W9-ARZ-436

MANAGING THE COMMUNITY HOSPITAL:
SYSTEMS ANALYSIS OF A SWEDISH HOSPITAL

Managing the Community Hospital:

Systems Analysis of a Swedish Hospital

ERIC RHENMAN

*Professor of Business Administration,
University of Lund, Sweden
Senior fellow of the Scandinavian
Institutes for Administrative Research*

Translated from the Swedish by
JULIE SUNDQVIST

SAXON HOUSE | LEXINGTON BOOKS

ST. PHILIPS COLLEGE LIBRARY

© Copyright Eric Rhenman 1973

All rights reserved. No part of this publication may be reproduced, stored in a retrieval system, or transmitted in any form or by any means, electronic, mechanical, photocopying, recording, or otherwise without the prior permission of D. C. Heath Ltd.

Published by

SAXON HOUSE, D.C. Heath Ltd.
Westmead, Farnborough, Hants, England

Jointly with

LEXINGTON BOOKS, D. C. Heath & Co.
Lexington Mass. U. S. A.

First published in Swedish as

*Centrallasarettet. Systemanalys
av ett svenskt sjukhus,*

Studentlitteratur, Lund 1969

ISBN 0 347 01022 9
LC No. 73-5249

Printed in Great Britain by
Kingprint Limited, Richmond, Surrey

Contents

v

47458

Foreword to the Swedish Edition

The aims of the study

When beginning this work in February 1965, members of the research team had discussions with leading persons on the National Council for Hospital Rationalisation and the Central Board of Hospital Planning. It was agreed that a description of the business, economic, and organisational aspects of a Swedish hospital would be useful, among others, in the following contexts:

1 To stimulate ideas on different ways of rationalising hospital operations and to obtain an initial basis for evaluating the ways in which different measures aimed at rationalisation affect the hospital *as a whole*.

2 As a contribution to general knowledge of hospital administration.

3 To compare it with other types of organisations. (One of organisation theory's most important aims is the study of how differences in general environment, technology, size, etc. influence the administration of an organisation.)

4 As a case study for teaching purposes.

Except for the fact that while the study was in progress we found it difficult to distinguish between (1) and (2), the aims of this text remain unchanged.

The study in relation to other research

Most researchers who have studied hospitals have done so using terms of reference acquired outside the hospital. The reader is referred to some examples in the list of references which deal with anthropological, sociological and socio-psychological studies of hospitals. Thus, in planning this study, it was not possible for us to relate it to any generally accepted traditions in hospital research. Nor were we interested in this approach. In a few theoretical studies,[1] I had formulated certain terms of reference which I thought suitable for business economic organisation studies, i.e. for research aimed at increasing efficiency. We had also carried out a pilot case study of a textile industry[2] and were interested in continuing our research in completely different kinds of organisations. A savings bank and a hospital seemed to be suitable objects of study.[3]

In planning this study, we also had another reason for making it as different from others as possible; this concerned the balance between description and consulting. As is described in chapter 1, we thought it important not only to describe the hospital but to indicate how this study could be used to give advice and make decisions about desirable changes. During one phase of this investigation, I even had the intention of combining as one report an empirical study of how management consultants work and this study of a hospital, so that I could show how the methods of problem-solving used in practice and the research results of more recent organisation theory could be coordinated into an analysis and evaluation of an organisation. Unfortunately, these two reports were so extensive that this was impossible.[4]

Now that several years have passed since the study was planned, it is fairly natural that, in several respects, I feel removed from and critical of the terms of reference used. Bearing this in mind, I would like to point out some of my own reservations.

The hospital is an open, controlled production system. This means that the work of the hospital is highly dependent on variations and disturbances, both external and internal, and that it has administrative and control systems which try to counteract these disturbances and keep activities running more or less smoothly. Thus, in order to be able to evaluate the hospital's administration, it has to be set in relation to the demands of the environment and of the hospital's own production system. This, briefly, is the theoretical point of departure for this study.

Even after completion of the study, I still think that the concept of the hospital as an open, controlled production system enables us to understand and evaluate some of its most important problems. Since the hospital constitutes one of the most disturbed production systems imaginable, we who have participated in the project believe that we have learned a great deal, not only about hospitals, but about production and production control. But objections can, of course, be made to the approach which was chosen.

The most important objection can be attributed to the fact that I have become wholly convinced that it is easier to understand the problems in an organisation if a distinction is made between problems which arise due to variations and disturbances and those which are the result of more long-term structural changes.

There are special resources and methods in a hospital which are used to resist the disruptive effects of unpredictability or variations and disturbances. Changes in work tempo and the quality of treatment are examples of ways that variations in workload and disturbances can be counteracted (see Table 7.3).

However, these resources and methods of handling variations and uncertainty can be used to cope with changes only up to a point. If certain limits are exceeded and if changes exist for a long period of time (or forever), completely new problems of adaption arise. Figures 1 and 2 distinguish between recurring and non-recurring changes.

In dealing with changes in this study of what we shall call General Hospital in Industry Town, we have not treated non-recurring changes in depth. My general (mainly intuitive) impression of the hospital is that it handles variations and disturbances quite admirably, regardless of whether they originate in the environment (e.g. as variations in patient flow) or within the hospital (e.g. unexpected complications in treatment of a patient). On the other hand, there is reason to question whether the hospital has the ability to handle certain structural changes quickly enough. Examples include changes required because of an increase in the need for medical care; medical progress; variations in the labour market; and growing controversy between what it is medically and economically possible to achieve in medical care.

The difficulty of distinguishing between variations and disturbances caused by structural changes is so much the more serious because, in all probability, we lack suitable terms of reference to describe structural

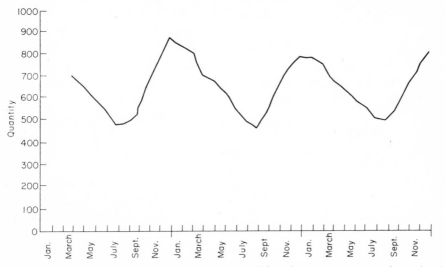

Fig. 1   Recurring changes can be dealt with using resources and methods inherent in the existing structure.

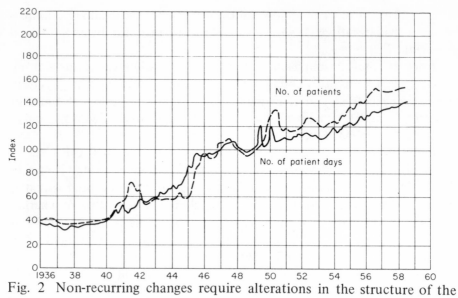

Fig. 2 Non-recurring changes require alterations in the structure of the hospital.

changes in the environment and in the hospital. Studies of other organisations which I have reported on[5] have shown that the most difficult adaption problems result from changes in values in the environment and the subsequent demands for change in the organisation's own value system. Increased demand and expanding medical specialisation require changes in the hospital, although methods already exist for solving these problems: more beds and more outpatient departments. But how should changed values be handled—changes such as re-examination of views on life or death, or who should have to wait for whom in a hospital, or the weighing of economic aspects against others, or the boundaries between medical care and social welfare service?

A study such as this depends to a large extent on the way that the researcher decides to define the system under investigation. A sound rule is to try to extract a system which is as self-contained as possible. This is because overdependence on the surrounding environment makes it difficult to understand internal conditions in an organisation unless a careful description of the environment is included (and this would, in fact, imply altering the boundaries of the system). In retrospect, we are able to claim that even though the hospital is 'fenced in', it is still a very open system and that studies of a clinical department or the county council would in all probability have provided us with a system possessing more definite boundaries.

xii

The emergence of the report

The preliminary phases of the study are described in chapter 3, mainly to give the reader an opportunity of becoming acquainted with the hospital as we experienced it during the first few months of this study. The subsequent collection of data and compilation of reports is a long story of the researcher's trials and tribulations. It did not take us long to discover that the hospital did not contain much of the data we were used to finding in firms, e.g. full financial accounts, production statistics and organisational handbooks. There were also large differences between the hospital and industrial firms in other respects. Many of the factors we were most interested in, such as disturbances and variations and the ways in which these were controlled, were in many instances more complex than in a commercial firm. Our task became even more difficult once we realised that the hospital's own definition of its administration was much too narrow, mainly because the doctors and nurses were the ones who actually performed the most important administrative tasks, such as diagnosis and planning.

The collection of data constantly required new methods of measurement, and though everyone at the hospital was more than willing to help us with all kinds of possible and impossible 'measurements', we sometimes could not avoid having to repeat collection of certain data before those aspects which seemed interesting could be described in full. One possible result of this process is that the report might be particularly valuable as a source of reference for those engaged in studies of hospitals.

This report would certainly have never come about without the constant stimulation we derived from the various parties involved. We had the opportunity to discuss drafts of the report during long conferences with leading employees and representatives of the county council, the hospital director, the chief nurse, and the department chiefs' association at General Hospital. In the spring of 1967, about thirty experts were invited to a seminar arranged by the Association of County Councils and the National Council for Hospital Rationalisation. These discussions, which involved deliberations as to changes that, at least experimentally, should be made at General Hospital and other hospitals, were extremely stimulating.

A preliminary mimeographed report was distributed in the spring of 1966 and another version prepared for the seminar. We decided to postpone this final publication, primarily because it did not seem suitable to distribute the report until we could claim complete anonymity for the hospital with a clear conscience. In fact, the hospital described no longer exists. The conditions at General Hospital have changed in many respects since this report was written.

Views in further research

This study of General Hospital has been especially useful to the Swedish Institute for Administrative Research because it has provided many ideas for further research. I will briefly mention a few of them as well as some general suggestions for Swedish hospital research which have emerged from a recent study trip to the United States.

A Swedish social science researcher, especially, perhaps, a business economic researcher, is used almost always to being at a disadvantage in comparison with American colleagues. In business economics this is not only due to the comparatively larger resources at the Americans' disposal and a long tradition of cooperation between firms and universities. An equally important factor is that many phenomena and objects of study — large firms, professional executives, active marketing, automation, electronic data processing, ect.—became available in American society first. The Swedish researcher, and to an even greater extent those in other European countries, often have to follow up pioneering American studies several years later.

We, in Sweden, have the possibility of attaining a key position in the field of hospitals. Large general and regional hospitals, planned medical and health care, redistribution of roles within the hospital and coordination of medical care, public health and social welfare activities are all phenomena being discussed and experimented with in the USA, whereas we are already putting them into practice. The extent of social science research in the USA has, of course, resulted in a number of very valuable studies of hospitals specialising in either physical medicine or mental illness. Contractual research institutes, consulting firms, and to some extent, academic researchers continue pursuing these studies, but my impression is that the orientation and planning of them is disrupted because, politically speaking, society is not ready to make drastic interventions in American medical care and because there are so many more controversial and neglected research areas. Thus, many researchers who used to be interested in health and medical care now seem to be in the process of turning to areas such as urgent urban problems.

Now that the development and rationalisation of the resources of the government and the Association of County Councils have been coordinated, we in Sweden should also be able to begin an extensive programme. The growing interest of the real specialists in this area – the doctors and nurses – in more general issues such as hospital administration, combined with an increase in the educational qualifications of social scientists should make it possible to recruit qualified personnel for these tasks. I hope that those engaged in this work will be able to avoid repeating the mistakes which were made in research in economics and industrial sociology.

Time and motion studies and traditional rationalisation in hospitals can yield some results, but are not, in themselves, particularly important. Nor can better accounting methods, simplified administrative routines, budget systems, and other instruments for economic control have a significant effect when it comes to solving these problems, unless they are used in a much wider context. Attitude surveys among personnel, aimed at finding out the effects of different kinds of leadership or organisational arrangements, turn out to be a blind alley, just as they were in industrial firms.

Instead, we have no choice but to accept that medical care is a complex system and that we know nothing about it as an entity because we are only acquainted with isolated elements or subsystems. Of course a research programme has to involve some kind of division of labour and boundaries have to be set for individual projects. But this should occur on the basis of acceptance of the fact that it is the entity which is important. Medical care and social welfare functions for the surrounding society have to be studied as the highest level in a research programme. On the next systems level, knowledge about conditions of dependency between the various components in medical care and social welfare is an important, and almost completely neglected, task. Other essential levels–if we limit ourselves to medical care–include studies of county councils, medical units, clinical departments, and nursing units. I would also like to maintain that a detailed study of the smallest but most important components constitutes another of the most neglected tasks. The doctor's role in solving medical problems, and in decision making in particular, should be understood much more clearly before studies of large units can be interpreted. General descriptive models have to be developed before this research on different systems levels can be coordinated.

Of course, all this might seem to be an impossible task because of its scope. But I would like to contend that this is the only feasible way and that the work should be planned in cycles so that the models can be refined on each system's level with respect to the results obtained on adjacent levels and in conjunction with methodological developments.

Division of work and financing

When the original research grant for this project was approved, the National Council for Hospital Rationalisation appointed an advisory committee in the autumn of 1964. The members of the committe were Bertil Jacobson, Rune Lind, Sten Troedsson, the director of the county council under study, and the director at General Hospital. Bertil Jacobson later resigned from the committee and was replaced by Gunnar Biörck and Stig Lindgren. This group worked in a very informal—and therefore even more useful—way. Most of all, the members of the group scrutinised plans and drafts of reports. I also received similar support from many others such as Åke Asplund, Gillis Claus, Peter Heimann, Gunnar Högberg, S. Åke Lindgren, Gösta Lyttkens, and Karl-Erik Westlund. In the planning stage, Hans Westholm devoted nearly a week to helping us understand the first principles of the hospital. This help, and lengthy discussions with Gunnar Biörck and Gunnar Högberg, enabled us to progress in our work. During the planning and initiation of the study, I received vital assistance from Professor Thomas Thorburn. Among my other colleagues at the Stockholm School of Economics, Professor Gunnar Westerlund, Professor Paulsson Frenckner, and Edgar Borgenhammar provided valuable ideas and impulses.

Even if I, as author, assume complete responsibility for the final version of this report, I have to confess the degree to which I have depended on my colleagues at the Swedish Institute for Administrative Research (SIAR). After working on the project for a number of months, several of them vowed that they would never again devote themselves to organisation research—at least not with me—but fortunately they revoked such vows. Roger Wallis, Christer Wallroth, and Curt Berg helped in collecting data during the first year. Carl-Johan Lindblad went to live in Industry Town for several months and resided alternately as 'patient' in the 'old nursing home' and as 'nurse' in various flats which were temporarily vacant. Jan Edgren, Anne-Marie Jonsson, and Lennart Sjöberg helped me edit the final version.

Much to my embarrassment, guarantees of anonymity prevent me from giving a detailed account of our dependence on the hospital director, chief physician, chief nurse, director of the county council, and chairman of the executive committee. These individuals gave us unlimited access to documents in the hospital (including their personal files), and from the beginning, made our business their business. We have never worked in an organisation where we received so much help. The most admirable aspect is perhaps the way in which the department chiefs, junior doctors, nurses,

xvi

and other nursing personnel gave us their assistance by cooperating in interviews, filling in our questionnaires, and often compiling various statistics for us. Throughout the report there is almost never any discussion of non-response, for this was never a serious problem for us.

This project was financed mainly by grants from the National Council for Hospital Rationalisation and its successor, the National Institute for Planning and Rationalisation of Medical Care and Social Welfare. Parts of the study were financed by the Bank of Sweden Fund. The county council in question provided a small additional grant. The data processing was financed by a grant from the University of Lund. Certain additional costs were paid for by the Economic Research Institute at the Stockholm School of Economics and by the Swedish Council for Personnel Administration (PA-rådet). Despite all these grants, the project involved costs which the Swedish Institute for Administrative Research had to cover.

The laborious job of typing, coding interviews and questionnaires, calculations, and various kinds of controls was performed by SIAR's secretarial staff, particularly with the cooperation of Margareta Ericsson, Monica Ewerth, Eva Jonsson, Barbro Orrung, and Ulla Stymne.

Eric Rhenman
Stanford, California
July 1968

Notes

1 Rhenman, E., *The Organization—a Controlled System*, Stockholm 1966 (SIAR-1).
2 Berg, C., *et al. Bruksbolaget—Ett företags anatomi* (The Mill Company— The Anatomy of a Firm), FFI, PA-rådet, SAF, Stockholm 1965 (mimeograph).
3 Hellgren, C. *et al. Serviceföretaget—tre organisationsteoretiska synsätt* (the Service Firm—Three Different Organisational Theory Viewpoints), Stockholm 1968 (SIAR-S-15; mimeograph).
4 This study by management consultants is reported separately in E. Rhenman, *Organisationsplanering* (Organisational Planning), Läromedelsförlagen, Stockholm 1968 (SIAR-S-13).
5 Rhenman, E., *Organization Theory for Long-range Planning*, Wiley, London 1973 (SIAR-18).

Foreword to the English Edition

This book presents a different approach to the study of a hospital. The study was performed by a group of researchers in organisational development, none of whom had extensive knowledge of hospitals or hospital administration. Because of this, the terms of reference used may seem unusual to the reader well versed in the subject. The hospital under study is taken at face value as an enterprise and looked at to find the interactions which take place within and around it to produce a product. It is the source and extent of these interactions with which the study is concerned.

Administration itself is considered in its broadest sense as being the common thread which binds together essentially separate but interdependent activities. Administration does not even have to be done by an administrator; anybody who interacts purposefully participates in the administrative process according to this concept. Thus, when physicians and nurses make medical decisions concerning patient care they are participating in the hospital's production administration. In my opinion doctors and nurses are important members of the management of a hospital because of their direct influence on the production process.

From a theoretical viewpoint this is a case study applying the 'principle of consonance' (Rhenman, 1973) or the 'contingency theory of organisation' (Lawrence and Lorsch, 1967). Its contribution is to suggest languages (Normann, 1972) which can be used to describe important sub-systems of an organisation in great detail. As such I think it can be regarded as something of a pioneer work.

Sweden has often been regarded as a forerunner in the provision of health care services. Perhaps the most characteristic feature of the Swedish health and medical system is that it is financed by taxes and a national health insurance programme (so often referred to as 'socialised'). The hospitals themselves are owned and operated by twenty-five local governmental bodies, the county councils. All the physicians working in the hospitals are full-time salaried staff, in other words not working on a fee for service basis. The Swedish state has a supervisory function and influences development mainly through legislation, research and education. The increased concern with rising costs has provided impetus to planning

xviii

and coordination efforts as well as attempts to provide care more efficiently. In these matters, the State has been trying to function as a catalyst to help the county councils in their efforts.

This book centres to a large extent on the physician's role (some Swedish readers have criticised the book because it concentrates too much on the doctor and too little on the other personnel categories found in the hospital). We look at the doctor as an employee, a supervisor, an upholder of medical standards, and an administrator and decision maker. That the central health and medical care authorities recognise the doctor's significant role is evidenced by the large number of recent reforms which apply specifically to him. The dichotomy between the doctor and administrator is starting to erode. The doctor can no longer sit on 'the clinical side of the house' and say that he does not participate in administration. The slowness in accepting this has been accompanied by a heavy increase in the number of administrative staff.

The foreword to the Swedish edition, which we recommend to the reader, stresses the importance of distinguishing between problems which arise due to short term variations and disturbances and those which are the result of more long range structural changes. Doubts are raised as to the hospital's ability to accomplish the structural changes required due to the increased need for medical care; that is, the increasing gap between what can be accomplished medically and what it is economically feasible to supply.

In translating this book into English, the question arose as to whether or not the text should be edited more or less extensively before the translation was made. The main reason for substantial editing was that the book had been written several years previously. As a result, statistics were no longer current, and certain situations no longer applied due to a number of changes which had been made in the Swedish health and medical care system.

Despite all this, the main reason why I refrained from altering the original text and instead described the most important changes in notes at the end of each chapter is not only a matter of resources, but perhaps more because I felt it would be difficult to make such sweeping changes and still retain the full character of the study.

In order to help the foreign reader, specifically Swedish conditions which were thought to require an explanation have been commented on in notes to the original text.

Julie Sundqvist translated the book. Fredrik von Bergen, who is well acquainted with American and Swedish health and medical care, checked the translation and pointed out those parts of the text which required clarification. Anne-Marie Jonsson, who also took part in the original study, compiled the notes. Inga-Britt Aggeklint and her staff performed the laborious task of typing the manuscripts. I extent my gratitude to all these persons.

Eric Rhenman
Stockholm, January 1973

1 Introduction

This report is a description and evaluation of a Swedish hospital from a business administration point of view. The study has three purposes. First, we would like to contribute a scientific basis for discussing the possibilities of improving administration and organisation in Swedish hospitals. Second, we want to formulate material for use in education in hospital administration. Third, we want to make a contribution to general organisation theory. This introductory chapter gives a detailed description of the background to each of these aims, and a survey of the report as a whole. Some 'advice to the reader' concludes this chapter.

A business administration approach to the hospital

Sweden's gross national product was slightly more than 100 billion Swedish Crowns[1] in 1965. An estimated 5 billion of this was used to provide health care services, i.e. care of the acutely, chronically and mentally ill, plus investments in hospital equipment, construction of new facilities, medical school costs, etc. This means that public health and medical care comprise a business sector larger than the Swedish iron and steel industry. In addition, this socioeconomic sector is growing very rapidly. The share of Sweden's gross national product allotted to health care has probably increased by about 40 per cent in the last decade. Thus, the provision of these services is the object of considerable attention. Many questions are being asked as to what can be done to use available resources in the best possible way. However, this type of discussion is not merely a Swedish phenomenon. Public health and medical care is also a vital issue in most European countries and the USA. The debate in Sweden has become particularly intense because many people are highly critical and are beginning to demand radical changes.[2] During the past few years, the mass media have involved the general public in this debate.

Criticism of the current situation centres around two major aspects. Some critics maintain that health care does not receive sufficient resources. Those responsible for providing the population with medical care have been accused of stinginess and neglect, resulting in an acute shortage of health and medical personnel.[3] Increased and improved education and

1

training of personnel—doctors, as well as nurses and other paramedical personnel—and measures that could stimulate recruitment, such as salary increases, day care centres for children, and tax benefits, are advocated. Other critics claim that increases in personnel are not sufficient, or even the most suitable way of coping with the 'crisis in medical care'. They feel that the health care sector lags behind other parts of society in terms of effectiveness and should thus be made more rational.

This so-called ineffectiveness is attributed to numerous causes. Many proposals have been made for increasing effectiveness. Some have had to do with basic issues in the organisation of the health care sector,[4] such as the reallocation of resources between in- and out-patient care,[5] or the coordination of health and social welfare activities. Other proposals concern more limited but important changes in various areas such as methods of serving and feeding patients, the daily routine in hospitals, doctors' access to paramedical personnel, specialisation in hospitals, the internal organisation of departments, the top management of hospitals, medical schools, coordination and distribution of work among different personnel groups, and the system of charges and fees.

These examples indicate that many of the proposals are related to hospital administration and organisation. Several of the issues remind us of earlier discussions with regard to the organisation and administration of industrial firms. The debate about recruiting hospital administrators, and their education and status, corresponds to a similar discussion about the recruitment, education and role of business executives. Business administration literature for line-staff deals with questions not unlike those recurring in discussions of the doctors' status in the hospital. The debate on 'democracy in the hospital' has many similarities to the debate on 'industrial democracy' that has been in progress for several decades. The status of personnel specialists in the hospital is currently being debated, while a corresponding question was topical in industrial firms about fifteen years ago. Many similar examples could be given.

As for efforts to alleviate the deficiencies, at least one group has applied experience, methods, and practices from industry and used these to establish guidelines. These guidelines include special instruments for rationalisation developed for industry, e.g. time and motion studies and methods for organising, planning, coordinating, and controlling work. The following quotations illustrate this approach:

> We should try as hard as possible to extend our perspective of an almost revolutionary development that will probably continue for a long time. I think the situation today makes it natural to apply

2

experience from industry and private business where the possibilities for overcoming situations forced upon us for various reasons are completely different.[6]

There are health care analogies to many of the tasks that have been rationalised in industry. Other tasks specific to public health and medical care have to be studied as entities, but there is no doubt that savings can be achieved by using modern methods of industrial rationalisation. These kinds of rationalisation are already in progress at some hospitals and have yielded good results. But efforts thus far are insignificant when compared to those in industry. There is probably no exaggeration in the statement that public health and medical care constitute an almost untouched area from the point of view of rationalisation. The solution to personnel and cost problems in health care requires efforts that are thirty or forty times greater than those being made at present.[7]

Public health and medical care have become powerful factors in society: not only do they cost billions, but they have also created a powerful administrative apparatus. We have to be constantly aware of over-organisation, administrative tyranny, monetary waste, and tendencies towards impersonal and mechanised care of human beings. Health care has been compared to an industry. The comparison is justified and there are obvious similarities, but the differences—not the similarities—are the most important. Nothing is more erroneous than the way hospital administrators regard hospitals as industries and evaluate the effectiveness of hospitals according to industrial yardsticks. The upper limit for rationalisation has already been reached and exceeded. Where are we headed?[8]

Education of hospital administrators

If we use the term 'hospital administrator' in a collective sense to designate hospital directors and managers (generally, doctors practising within the hospital), there are about 100 such administrators in Sweden today. This study reveals that there is reason to believe that the efficiency of a hospital depends primarily on the administrative ability of individual department heads, of whom there are about 1,000 in Sweden at this time. Recently, the need for education and training in hospital administration has been shown to extend far beyond these two groups.

3

Education of doctors is not really aimed at their obligation to handle medical care advantageously from an economic point of view. Medical students do not receive any instruction in administration or any of the tasks which are the responsibility of the hospital administrator.[9]

Our account of the education of hospital administrators in the USA implies that Sweden, with a complete lack of this kind of education, seems almost like an under-developed country in this area. It is imperative that some Swedish form of education in hospital administration be created.[10]

A number of initiatives have been taken and others are being prepared.[11] Several of the commissions that have initiated or begun to plan education in hospital administration have been in contact with us. We have a clear impression that one of their most significant difficulties is related to the lack of educational material and realistic examples and case studies from the hospital world. Contacts with American physicians and researchers in this area have shown that conditions are to some extent the same in the USA. 'We have to use examples from engineering industries, the construction industry, oil companies and railroads, in educating hospital administrators,' says a professor at a well-known American university.[12]

Obviously, many different kinds of educational material are required, primarily perhaps the traditional Harvard-type case studies.[13] But relatively easily comprehensible scientific descriptions of hospitals are probably equally important. They can be used as a basis for problem-oriented discussions that provide the student with a scientific frame of reference and a method of analysis which he can use in new situations. An important purpose of this report is to present this kind of description of a Swedish hospital using a business administration approach.

The development of organisation theory

The primary task of the theory of business administration is to support business executives and other leaders who make decisions about the management of firms and other organisations. The assumption is usually made that top management aims at the greatest possible effectiveness. Researchers in this area have often formulated their task in terms of finding 'the most effective administration or organisation'. In any case,

4

this was the goal that classical organisation theorists set themselves, and many of their successors have tried to formulate principles for effective administration. Two sets of principles are compared in Table 1.1.

But these principles have been criticised from several standpoints. They are said to have been formulated so generally that they do not serve any purpose. The empirical basis has also been questioned, and the opposite principles have sometimes been claimed to be equally valid. As a whole, this line of research has now been abandoned. The mistakes made in trying to formulate these kinds of principles seem to have been as follows:

1 Assumptions were made on the basis of oversimplified ideas about how the firm and its management functioned.
2 The large differences between different firms were not taken into account.
3 The concept of effectiveness was either unclearly or erroneously defined.

At least as far as these three points are concerned, more recent research has tried new approaches. Descriptions of the industrial firm and its management have become more varied and a number of concepts and assumptions have been introduced of which members of the older school were unaware. Attempts have been made to determine the differences between different commercial firms and organisations. Researchers have tried to develop a theory which can explain and predict the firm's goals. All this has provided a basis for specifying concept of effectiveness.[14]

But this development has had little or no influence on professional managers. The wide gap between the description and analysis of organisational conditions by modern teachers of organisation theory and that made by experienced practitioners was clearly shown in a series of laboratory experiments which I carried out, and in which highly experienced and even relatively well-read managers were asked to solve concrete organisational problems.[15]

My conclusion from these experiments was primarily that more recent research results have to be reformulated and reassembled to be more applicable to the problem-solving techniques that managers have to use. This reformulation is required so long as research cannot provide better techniques. Similar results are reported in *Approaches to Organizational Design*,[16] by Cyert and March,[17] and by Rubenstein and Haberstroh.[18] It therefore seems that a very important aim of research must be to show how the manager's methods of problem solving and the research results from modern organisation theory can be coordinated in an analysis

5

TABLE 1.1

Organisational principles: 1916 and 1961

Organisational principles Fayol (1916)[19]	Organisational principles Stieglit (1961)[20]
1 The organisation has to be adapted to the firm's aims, assets, and needs.	*Objectives* 1 The objectives of the enterprise and its component elements should be clearly defined and stated in writing. The organisation should be kept simple and flexible.
2 Distribution and delegation of authority and responsibility are required.	
3 Authority and responsibility go hand in hand.	
4 Discipline is absolutely necessary to the success of the firm.	*Activities and grouping of activities* 2 The responsibilities assigned to a position should be confined as far as possible to the performance of a single leading function.
5 An individual should never receive orders from more than one manager with regard to carrying out a definite task.	3 Functions should be assigned to organisational units on the basis of homogeneity of objective to achieve the most efficient and economic operation.
6 Only one manager should be responsible for the execution of a distinct goal.	
7 The degree of centralisation is determined by the situation.	*Authority* 4 There should be clear lines of authority running from the top to the bottom of the organisation, and accountability from bottom to top.
8 It is wrong to deviate from the usual official channels if there are no good reasons for doing so, but it is even worse to adhere to them if damage to the firm is involved.	5 The responsibility and authority of each position should be clearly defined in writing.
9 'One job for every individual and every individual at his job'.	6 Accountability should always be coupled with corresponding authority.
10 The organisation should provide possibilities for systematic planning, good coordination, and adequate control.	7 Authority to take or initiate action should be delegated as close to the scene of action as possible.
	8 The number of levels of authority should be kept to a minimum.
	Relationships 9 There is a limit to the number of positions that can be effectively supervised by a single individual.
	10 Everyone in the organisation should report to only one supervisor.
	11 The accountability of higher authority for the acts of its subordinates is absolute.

6

and evaluation to determine whether the administration of a hospital, for instance, is suitably designed.

The study

We have tried to accomplish the above three aims of this study by setting it up as follows. In accordance with a fundamental proposition (generally accepted by top management and now being acknowledged by researchers), we begin the analysis with a basic description of the hospital and its environment. This is organised in terms of a description of the external forces affecting the hospital (the hospital's participant relations, chapter 4) and the activity for which the hospital was created, i.e. the care and treatment of patients (the hospital's production, chapter 5). Applying organisation theory propositions about the relation between an industrial firm's situation and the demands on its administration, we then formulate a number of expected demands on the hospital's administration (chapters 6 and 7). Next, we study the hospital's administration as it really is (chapters 6 and 7). By comparing real conditions with the demands formulated earlier, we can evaluate the hospital's administration. In conclusion, this evaluation is used as a basis for some proposals for improving the hospital's administration (chapter 8).

Chapter 2 contains a more precise formulation of our theoretical assumptions. The reader who is neither interested in, nor familiar with, the literature on organisation theory should be able to skip this chapter. On the other hand, the report of our first visit to General Hospital (chapter 3) should perhaps be of interest as an introduction to the hospital described in this study.

Advice to the reader

To hospital administrators, doctors, nurses, and others primarily interested in our first and second aims

A business administration approach is used in this study. This means that the report contains many terms commonly used in business administration. We hope that our definitions of unusual and unfamiliar terms in the text will facilitate understanding. We also hope that you will find it worthwhile to become acquainted with some of the concepts of business administration. At this stage, we would like to warn you about the word

7

'administration'. Here are some of the ways in which staff at General Hospital defined this term:

Administration is all the tasks that do not have anything to do with the patient.
Administration is all desk and office work.
Administration is bureaucracy, rules, laws, regulations, and norms.
Administration is the people who work in the yellow building.
Administration is the director of the hospital and his staff.

Administration means something completely different in this report. It is formally defined on page 16 (see also page 219). More simply (but not fully satisfactorily), we use 'administration' to signify decision making and control. The job of administrators is to make decisions and to control.

We hope that this reminder about the meaning of 'administration' will help readers to discard any ideas about this term which resemble those in the statements quoted above.

To organisation experts, management researchers, and others primarily interested in our third aim

You may be surprised that we chose a hospital as a model for testing and demonstrating a method of evaluating administration. Would it not have been more suitable to select a 'regular' firm as our object of study? There are several answers to this question. Of course, the three aims we mentioned were the decisive motive for not being able to select an industrial firm as our object of study. In addition, early in the planning stages there were several arguments in favour of choosing a hospital for an organisation theory study. These reasons became increasingly important as the study progressed. First, it was clear from the beginning that the hospital was, in many respects, a very open organisation and easily accessible for studies. We expected cooperation with doctors to be difficult;[21] on the contrary, during our first visit we found that most were eager to support us, and we discovered a number of advantages in the choice of a hospital for our study. Second, due to the large number of university graduates and other experts, the existence of complex technology, several different public welfare goals, a board of trustees less powerful than boards in industrial firms, we felt that in some respects the hospital could teach us something about future problems in industrial firms.[22] Third, with regard to the hospital's administration, there were certainly many viewpoints—and

8

often completely opposing opinions—even among the experts. This implied that anyone making an evaluation of the administration's efforts would really have to take a stand on a number of conflicting issues.

Thus, this report should be regarded as a study of an industrial firm; certainly, an unusual kind of firm, but a very interesting one.

To all readers

A wise researcher once claimed that any good report on a research project should be able to be read as a travelogue. We hope that this report will fulfil this requirement in some respects. This exploratory journey has not carried us far in terms of miles or hours. But for those of us whose experience is mostly related to organisations other than hospitals, this has been a journey to a very foreign culture. We hope that all readers will become aware of, and share, the attitude we tried to adopt from the beginning—respect for the unknown. Even when we meet and describe conditions that seem irrational, or 'worse' in some other respect, than the conditions we are accustomed to in industrial firms, we have tried to maintain a respectful attitude. Our collective impression is that a Swedish hospital is an impressive organisation which can learn from other organisations, including industrial firms, but which also has something to teach them.

Notes

[1] In 1965, one US dollar was equivalent to 5.165 Swedish crowns and one pound sterling to 14.435. Figures quoted throughout the text refer to Swedish crowns (cr.).

[2] In the past, medical care was paid for without giving priority to any particular cost category. Today, there is a new awareness of the necessity for grading public expenses, including those in the health care sector. According to the central authorities, psychiatry, long-term care and out-patient care are given priority over other medical areas in terms of investments in construction, and the allocation of physicians.

[3] The number of admissions to institutions for the education of doctors and other medical personnel increased considerably during the 1960s. The number of persons admitted to medical schools in Sweden increased from about 400 per year in 1965 to nearly 1,000 in 1971.

[4] Certain changes in medical care legislation were enacted in 1971 to augment the effectiveness of the medical care organisation and to increase

9

the degree of integration between in-patient and outpatient care.

[5] The 'seven-crown reform' is described in note 4 to chapter 4. One of the main purposes of this reform was to eliminate certain elements in the previous fee system which sometimes made it financially advantageous to the patient to be hospitalised rather than treated as an outpatient.

[6] Berg, O., 'Synpunkter på sjukhusadministration' (Views on Hospital Administration), *Sjukhuset 40*, 7 August 1963, p. 155.

[7] Malmström, S., 'Uttalande vid Svenska Sjukhusföreningens' Årsmöte 1962 (Excerpts from the Annual Meeting of the Swedish Hospital Association), *Svenska Sjukhusföreningens årsbok* 1962. Halmstad 1963, p. 77.

[8] Heymann, P., *Bättre sjukvård* (Improved medical care), Aldus/Bonniers, Stockholm 1964, p. 37.

[9] Biörck, G., 'Skämt åsido eller doktorn har inte tid' (All Kidding Aside or The Doctor Doesn't Have Time), *Svenska Läkartidningen 61* (1964): 14, p. 1144.

[10] Borgenhammer, E., and Otterland, A., 'Sjukvårdsadministratörernas utbildning' (Educating Hospital Administrators), *Svenska Läkartidningen 61* (1964): 18, p. 1480.

[11] A committee of the Association of County Councils has formulated a proposal for educating medical personnel and civil servants in hospital administration. Beginning in 1973, experimental courses in hospital administration will be taught at certain Swedish universities as part of a series of 'direct professionally oriented courses'.

[12] Notes from conversations with Professor Leroy K. Young, MD, Cornell University, Ithaca, New York 1966.

[13] Berg, C., *Case Studies in Organizational Research and Education*, (SIAR-10. mimeograph), Stockholm 1967.

[14] This development was described in more detail in E. Rhenman, *Industrial Democracy and Industrial Management*, (SIAR-8), van Gorcum & Comp., Assen 1968, and in E. Rhenman and B. Stymne, *Företagsledning i en föränderlig värld* (Management in a Changing World), Aldus, Stockholm 1965.

[15] Rhenman, E., *Organisationsplanering* (Organisational Planning) (SIAR-S-13), Läromedelsförlagen, Stockholm 1968.

[16] Buck, V. E., *et al.* 'A Model for Viewing an Organization as a System of Constraints' in Thompson, J. D. (ed.), *Approaches to Organizational Design*, University of Pittsburgh Press, Pittsburgh 1966.

[17] Cyert, R. M., and March, J. G., *A Behavioral Theory of the Firm*, Prentice-Hall, Englewood Cliffs N. J., 1963.

[18] Rubenstein, A. H., and Haberstroh, C. J., *Some Theories of Organization*, Irwin-Dorsey, Homewood Ill., 1964.

10

[19] Fayol, H., *Industriell och allmän administration* (Industrial and General Administration), Norstedts, Stockholm 1950 (1916).

[20] Stieglitz, H., *Corporate Organization Structures,* Studies in Personnel Policy, no. 83, *National Industrial Conference Board*, New York 1961.

[21] Perrow, C. 'Hospitals: Technology, Structure and Goals' in J. G. March (ed.), *Handbook of Organizations,* Rand McNally, Chicago 1965. This notes that many researchers have experienced this problem. Our advisers in central hospital agencies also indicated that this could become a serious problem.

[22] See the future outlook for industrial firms described, for example, by K. E. Boulding, 'The Future Corporation and Public Attitudes' in J. W. Riley (ed.), *The Corporation and its Publics*, Ardsley-on-Hudson N. Y., 1963.

2 The Hospital - a Controlled Production System

The hospital as a production system[1] will be studied in this chapter: we are interested in the different kinds of contributions coming into the hospital and the services and other inducements offered by the hospital. The term 'participants' refers to individuals or groups that provide these contributions and receive these inducements (see Fig. 2.1).

But a study of the contributions and inducements alone does not suffice. The internal conditions of the hospital are also relevant. Therefore, we have also to describe the way in which contributions are trans-

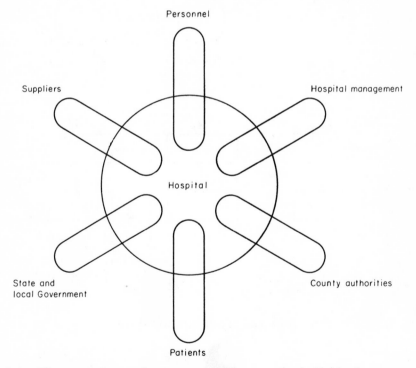

Fig. 2.1 The participants in an organisation are the individuals or groups that depend on it for the realisation of their personal goals, and on whom the organisation depends for its existence.[2]

13

formed into inducements. This is a complex process and, in order to achieve a fairly realistic description, we have to regard the hospital as a system of components that interact and influence one another in many different ways. There are various kinds of components. Some are productive, participating directly in the transformation of contributions into inducements. There are also administrative components in the hospital which process and transport information so that flows into and out of the hospital, and production within the hospital, are controlled (see Fig. 2.2).

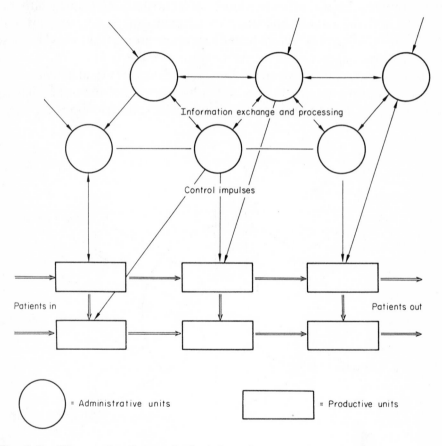

Fig. 2.2   The production and administration system.

Structure and behaviour

The first thing we want to describe in our study of the hospital is its

14

structure, i.e. its stable characteristics. Parts of the structure can be directly observed: for instance, the number of employees, the technical equipment, and the formally described organisation. As to other aspects, we can draw conclusions about the structure indirectly, by observing behaviour or processes. This can be exemplified by conclusions about actual lines of authority drawn on the basis of studies of who takes orders from whom. Much about the structure can also be learned from the interdependence of the productive components deduced from observations of the flows of information, material and patients between the components. We did not make many extensive studies of behaviour in the hospital. Instead, we interviewed members of the organisation, and often depended on their ability to draw conclusions as to structure from their observations of behaviour.

The concept of the structure of the hospital is very useful. We assume that if we know the structure and the external flows of material and information (i.e. from the participants), we can predict what will happen (the behaviour) within the hospital, at least for a short time.

We expect to find stability or some kind of structure in the ways in which the hospital relates to its participants within the production and administrative systems. When we talk about the participant system, the production system and the administration system, these are usually abbreviations for 'the structure of the hospital's participant system', 'the structure of the hospital's system' and 'the structure of the hospital's administrative system'. Later, these three systems in the hospital will be broken down even further. We will begin to talk about participant control and production control within the administration, which controls the flow into and out of the hospital, i.e. the flow of the hospital's participants. The latter is the part of the administration that controls production.

The stability exhibited by some of the components in an organisation, which we term its structure, is limited. Stability usually prevails only during a certain period of time, such as a day, a week, a year or a decade. Sometimes, our conception of stability during a certain period is only theoretical. In these instances, that which we call structure consists only of conditions which change more gradually than others. But the assumption that conditions are stable for a period is a practical simplification.

In any case, we expect the structure of the hospital to be more or less changeable for a relatively long time. If structural changes are irreversible, i.e. if the old structure does not return to its former state, changes are depicted as development. We assume that this development depends to a large extent on the hospital's administration. Therefore, a third subsystem of the administration can be called the development system.

15

Participant control
Production control
Development system
} Participant system
Productive system
Administration system
} Hospital

Fig. 2.3 Subsystems of the hospital.

Goals and effectiveness

The hospital's administration is a particularly important component. The administration is the person, or persons, primarily responsible to the various participants for the hospital's performance. We assume that this measurement of results is aimed primarily at evaluating whether the resources of the hospital have been used properly and whether the hospital has been able to maintain good relations with its various participants. Resources are contributions existing within the system that are at the direct disposal of the hospital management. Relations with a participant are a measure of the participant's willingness to continue to associate with the hospital.

One symptom of poor relations is exhibited when certain participants show dissatisfaction with the hospital. Patients can complain, via the press, or to the National Board of Health and Welfare. Dissatisfaction of personnel may be expressed by disloyalty or a high frequency of absenteeism. Poor relations between suppliers and the hospital may be expressed by unwillingness to make quick deliveries or offer other favours such as discounts. An even more serious symptom of poor relations is revealed when the participants begin to desert the hospital. This can eventually become a direct threat to its survival, and it may be forced to limit its activities to the extent that other hospitals assume its functions. In an extreme situation, the hospital might have to close.

Relations between an organisation and its participants usually depend on the way in which the inducements received by the participants are related to their demands or expectations. Since most organisations have a scarcity of such inducements, some symptoms of poor relations are a normal phenomenon. An organisation seldom has the ability to satisfy all its participants. This means that only the most serious symptoms of poor relations are perceived by the management as alarming.

16

Scarcity of inducements and effectiveness

The scarcity of inducements in an organisation such as a hospital can be affected in two different ways. First, the supply of inducements depends on the way in which an institution is run. Obviously, the greater the amount of inducements that can be produced by a given contribution, the less scarce they will be. Second, the supply of inducements is related to the conditions for exchanging contributions and inducements with the participants. The more the contributions that an organisation can obtain from its participants for a given quantity of inducements, without deterioration of relations, the less scarce the inducements will be.

We talk about an organisation's ability to gather and process contributions as its internal effectiveness and the expenditures which it has to make to secure these contributions from the participants as its external effectiveness.

Internal and external effectiveness depend on the structure of the organisation. In the short run, internal effectiveness depends on the production system and the structure of production control. External effectiveness in the short run depends on the participant system and the structure of participant control. Long-term external and internal effectiveness depend primarily on the development system. However, this study deals exclusively with short-term effectiveness.

Measurements of effectiveness in the hospital and its subsystems

It is impossible to determine whether an organisation such as a hospital has attained maximal effectiveness. Not even limited parts of the structure —such as the administration—can be evaluated in this way. But sometimes it is possible to determine whether one subsystem is superior to another. These evaluations cannot be performed separately because there are significant interdependencies between the environment in which an organisation operates and the effectiveness of its system. Participants' demands and power, available technology and norms, values and attitudes in the surrounding society are particularly important factors in the environment. In addition, there are important interdependencies that affect the effectiveness of different systems.

If we were to say that one subsystem A, is more efficient than an alternative, B, —for example, in combining several clinical departments into a bloc under a single chief instead of having completely independent departments—we are expressing something complex in a simplified way.

17

In other words, the hospital's effectiveness would increase if A replaced B, provided that other systems and the hospital's environment were not altered simultaneously.

Demands of the situation on the hospital's administration

It is often difficult to compare the efficiency of two subsystems when both are 'acceptable'. It is usually easier to determine whether a subsystem is relatively inefficient, i.e. whether there is at least one alternative structural design which, in a given situation, would increase the effectiveness of the organisation. A given situation also refers to the environment and structure of other subsystems. Since we are primarily interested in evaluating the administration's effectiveness, this could be formulated as follows: the environment, chosen strategy, and the production system all place certain demands on the administration so that the evaluation is aimed at determining whether the administration meets these demands.[3] For example, in an environment with large variations in demand and production facilities which do not allow for stocking of finished products, an administration that can control the participants so that variations in demand are reduced is superior to one lacking these characteristics. In other words, the latter does not meet the demands of the situation.

Comparing a hospital with other organisations

The close interdependence of different subsystems, and of the organisation and its environment, implies that comparisons between a hospital and industrial firms cannot be used as a basis for evaluating the hospital's effectiveness. Since the most important element involves adapting a subsystem to the demands of the situation, differences between the administration of the hospital and an industrial firm can be expected. But this is not to say that the hospital should be regarded as inefficient. Thus, the sense of making any comparisons at all becomes questionable.

On the other hand, business executives often channel a great deal of their interest into comparisons of different firms, and in particular, their management. Researchers have also studied these kinds of comparisons. In addition to the insight obtained with regard to the differences between various situations, comparisons are justifiable as a source of new ideas.

Earlier, we discarded the notion that we can evaluate whether an organisation has attained maximum effectiveness. We said that the only

18

possible and meaningful comparisons are those between different sub-systems. Comparisons with other organisations are often likely to provide ideas for new alternatives in terms of setting up a subsystem such as a new procedure, planning methods, or ways of organising research and development. These kinds of comparisons are probably especially valuable for an organisation in a changing environment. Environmental changes usually require development of an organisation's structure. Comparisons with other organisations already existing in a similar environment can provide many new ideas.

Notes

[1] This arose from one of the first empirical studies made by SIAR (Swedish Institute for Administrative Research). The theoretical framework was relatively incomplete but has since been more fully developed. For a more complete description of the theory see E. Rhenman, *Organization Theory for Long-range Planning* (SIAR-18), Wiley, London 1973.

[2] Rhenman, E., *Industrial Democracy and Industrial Management*, (SIAR-8), Assen: van Gorcum & Comp., Assen 1968.

[3] This can be seen as a special case of the 'principle of consonance' or the 'principle of fit'. See E. Rhenman, *Organization Theory for Long-range Planning* (SIAR-18), Wiley, London 1973, and P.R. Lawrence and J.W. Lorsch, *Organization and Environment. Managing Differentiation and Integration.* Harvard University, Boston 1967.

3 Choice of Hospital, a First Visit and Execution of the Study

Introductory considerations

One of the most important decisions to be made when planning this study was the choice of hospital. We viewed our study in two different ways: first, as part of our process of developing a method for describing and evaluating an organisation, and second, as a contribution to the debate on rationalising hospitals and health care. Thus, we were faced with conflicting requirements. The most important were that

1   The hospital should be reached easily from our normal place of work.
2   The county authorities, management, and personnel of the hospital should be positively inclined towards a scientific study of the hospital.
3   The hospital should have a reputation for being well run and have a fairly modern organisation.
4   The hospital should be medium-sized and 'typical' in other respects.

These criteria were a great help the first time we tried to sort out a number of potential objects for study. But no systematic selection was made on the basis of these criteria. We defined 'medium-sized' as 500–1,000 beds. Despite their location, none of the city or county hospitals in the Stockholm area seemed suitable.[1] These hospitals are so integrated that the object of study would have been difficult to define. Nor was it easy to specify the requirement that the hospital be 'typical'. Burling, Lentz, and Wilson[2] reported the same kinds of difficulties in choosing an object. The criteria they indicate are that the object should be an acute general hospital offering medical and surgical care, and that most patients should stay at the hospital for only a short time. Dunham and Weinberg[3] designate Columbus State Hospital (in Ohio) as 'representative' or typical among state mental hospitals. They supported this by comparing Columbus State Hospital with twelve neighbouring hospitals, and found that it was typical in its high usage rate and representative range of specialities.

Choice of hospital and our introduction

Before we could produce a systematic basis for decision, an energetic adviser to the central public health authorities had contacted the manage-

21

ment of General Hospital in Industry Town. From what we could gather with respect to location, size, facilities, range of specialties, organisation, and general reputation, there was nothing to disqualify this hospital. It was about sixty miles from Stockholm, had approximately 1,000 beds, fifteen clinical departments and a modern organisation. The administration consisted of a director and a chief of medical staff. In addition, a new system of nurse supervisors, recommended by the Association of Swedish County Councils, had recently been introduced. Instead of continuing our selection procedure we decided to make a pilot study. What follows is an account of the results of our first contacts with General Hospital, which took place at the end of 1964 and the beginning of 1965. In retrospect, with regard to representativeness, we draw the same conclusions as Dunham and Weinberg[4], that 'while we are perfectly aware that this contention is impressionistic we have found nothing that would argue against or detract from the hospital's representative character'.

During the course of our study, the director of the hospital or the chief of the medical staff usually introduced us personally to everyone we contacted. The director was very eager to help—either personally or through one of his assistants—with arrangements for our meetings with doctors on the medical staff. One Saturday morning, at a medical staff meeting, we had an opportunity to talk with around thirty doctors about our study, its background, and aims.

History of the hospital

General Hospital celebrated its fiftieth anniversary at the end of 1964. In connection with this celebration there was an exhibition depicting the history of the hospital and how it has expanded over the years. Various documents and interviews with, among others, a department chief who participated in compiling the hospital's history, gave us the following information.

The first hospital with a capacity of five beds was established in 1803 through private initiative. In 1914 the hospital was moved from the centre of town to its present location. A school of nursing has been affiliated with the hospital since 1925. The hospital was divided into different specialties in 1932. Development up to the present is shown in Figs. 3.1 and 3.2.

The number of employees increased from 40 to approximately 1,000 between 1916 and 1965, and the number of patient admissions from 1,750 to more than 15,000 per year.

22

Industry Town's hospital is called 'General Hospital'. This means that it is the largest hospital in the county and includes resources such as chest and rehabilitation clinics, a central laboratory, and departments of psychiatry and orthopaedics. Smaller, unspecialised county hospitals in Sweden do not have these facilities. Nevertheless, General Hospital in Industry Town is similar in some respects to Sweden's large regional hospitals (for instance with respect to its departmental structure).[5]

Owing to the hospital's high rate of growth, the demands on its administration have increased. Until 1960 a doctor had been in charge, assisted by a superintendent. In 1961 a hospital director, assisted by a physician (known as the chief of the medical staff) replaced the previous organisational set-up. In 1964 the nursing staff was reorganised, with a chief nurse and nursing supervisors replacing the matron and her assistants. The personnel department was expanded in 1964 to include the appointment of a personnel assistant. The position of special studies secretary was also established to assist the director and serve in a secretarial capacity for the Board of Trustees. A hospital accountant was appointed in 1965 to take

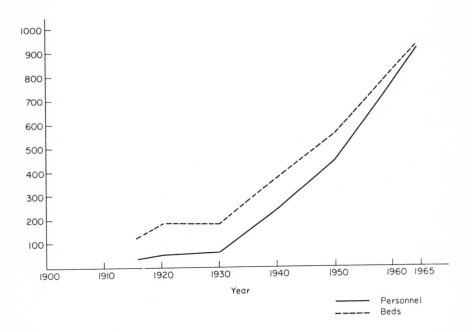

Fig. 3.1 Number of personnel and beds at General Hospital, 1914-1965.

23

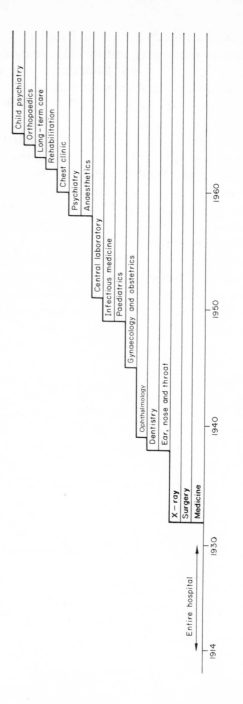

Fig. 3.2   Clinical departments at General Hospital, 1914-65.

24

charge of the financial section. And in 1966 the personnel department was expanded to include a personnel manager and an additional personnel assistant.

Size and resources

The preceding section gives some indication of the size and resources of the hospital. Later, in connection with our systematic study, we discovered that the hospital represents a strange mixture of small business and large organisation. With regard to the number of employees and volume of production, the hospital can be regarded as one of the largest 'firms' in Industry Town. It has approximately 1,000 employees, production is about 230,000 in-patient days and more than 100,000 outpatient visits.[6] The 'range of the product assortment' is indeed impressive. The rough classification used in the hospital's annual report indicates that it treats more than 2,000 different diseases in its in-patient units per year.

Two aspects of the hospital's resources that were easy to classify after our first visit were facilities and personnel. Figure 3.3 shows that the hospital is a conglomeration of the old and the new. An extension containing ten nursing units and several specialist units and clinical departments was opened as late as 1962. The oldest parts of the hospital include the surgery clinic and X-ray department, and date from 1914. There are difficulties to cope with in regard to the older parts of the hospital, particularly the department of infectious medicine. This department was originally a separate epidemic hospital which was assigned to General Hospital in 1949 (when the county took over its administration). It was integrated with the rest of the hospital as the department of infectious medicine in 1965. According to the county council (quoted in the hospital's personnel newspaper in 1964), construction of facilities for infectious diseases should have begun in 1964. At the time of our first visit, a shortage of resources still prevented execution of these plans.

There did not seem to be any acute crisis with respect to hospital facilities, but personnel conditions were much more serious. Because the hospital was fairly near Stockholm, it was probably easier to recruit qualified doctors for permanent positions than in other county hospitals, though understaffing of doctors was a serious problem in some departments. The situation with regard to nurses, auxiliaries, and orderlies was a much greater problem. The hospital was designated as the site of a strike planned by the Swedish Medical Association in 1964, but these plans never materialised. High employee turnover, and many vacancies, were

25

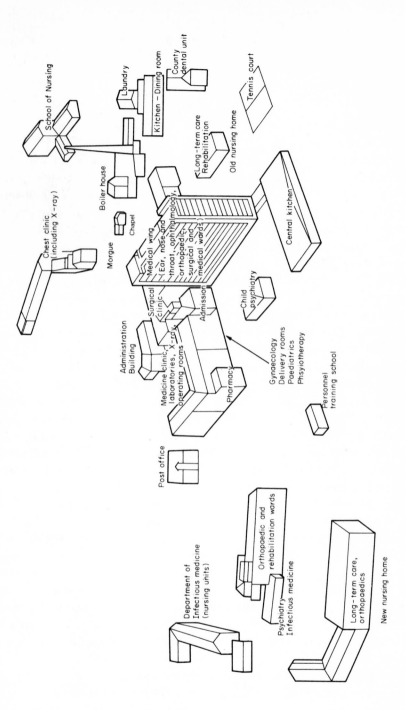

Fig. 3.3   General Hospital, 1965.

26

noted as the most serious problems. The hospital administration had recently hired a consultant to study various issues regarding personnel administration.

Formal organisation

The hospital's most recent improvements in organisation took effect on 1 October 1961, when the post of hospital director was established, and on 1 May 1964, when the new nursing supervisor organisation, recommended by the Association of County Councils, was introduced. These changes involved the appointment of a chief nurse and two (later on, three) nursing supervisors instead of the previous arrangement involving a matron and her assistants. The organisation chart shown in Fig. 3.4 was published in the hospital's personnel newspaper when these changes were introduced. Job descriptions were also written for most of the positions within the hospital's administration.

Our first study of the formal organisation included interviews with the hospital director, two department heads, the chief nurse, two charge nurses and the director's assistants, so that we could ascertain whether the actual role structure deviated from the formal structure. These interviews were highly unstructured. The interviewees were asked to tell about their jobs and the organisation they worked in. They were also given an opportunity to express their opinions about important problems.

The interviews gave us the impression that the hospital's board of trustees was less influential than the boards of directors in industrial firms that we had studied. One interviewee pointed out that:

> The board meets once a month. The meetings begin at 5 p.m. Since everyone wants to be home in time for supper they last no later than 6.30 p.m. This means that there is not much time for proper factual discussions. The funny thing is that all the department chiefs willingly paticipate in these meetings. This has its advantages but also means that the board members do not say very much. The real decisions are made in the executive committee, composed of the chairman and vice-chairman of the board, the chief of medical staff and the hospital director. It is rather indicative that these meetings often last more than five hours.

We also learned that the hospital's relations with the county council were good—which, according to a couple of interviewees, was to a large

27

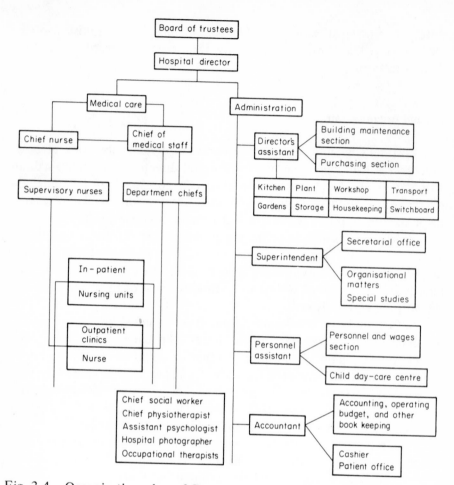

Fig. 3.4 Organisation plan of General Hospital in Industry Town.

extent attributable to the hospital director. His most important accomplishment, they said, had been in organising the administration at the hospital. The chief physician also commanded the respect of our interviewees. But the nursing supervisor organisation and the personnel department seemed to be in difficulty. These organisational units did not function as intended, partly due to a shortage of resources. It was implied, however, that this was a temporary problem.

There was one situation which our introductory interviews failed to reveal though it later turned out to be rather significant. Two of the largest clinical departments and the oldest service department were headed by doctors who would soon retire or who had been absent for long periods because of illness. It was surprising that we were not more concerned

28

about this situation during the planning stage. We observed rather quickly that these clinical departments were very important units and that, in many respects, the hospital could be regarded as a set of independent departments arranged in terms of mutual service components with certain common facilities.

So far as our study is concerned, it is difficult to evaluate the consequences of the periods during which the departments were without chiefs. But it seems likely that this situation greatly influenced relations between the department chiefs themselves and between the doctors and the hospital management as a whole. In retrospect we can only state that there appeared to be very good personal relations between members of the senior staff. 'Better than in most other places' was the opinion of several doctors who had recently joined the staff at General Hospital.

The nature of the hospital as 'common premises for a number of clinical departments' prompted us to clarify the dependency between and the conditions within departments. Most of all, we needed some simple charts to give us an idea of the patient and work flows. Figure 3.5 shows that the dependency between the various clinical departments was rather limited. Each specialty contained two highly independent 'production units', i.e. outpatient and in-patient care. The nursing units (of which the various specialties each had between one and four) took care of those patients who required hospitalisation for diagnosis and treatment.

Patients who came to the hospital during the day were examined and treated in the outpatient clinics. Since the doctors—particularly the department chiefs and some of their assistants—worked in both the in-patient and outpatient units, they were a unifying link within their specialties. The different service units joined the entire hospital together in the same way. Three of these, X-ray, the central laboratory, and the department of anaesthetics had their own department heads. Other service units, such as social workers, occupational therapists and physiotherapists, were incorporated in a less-clear way and seemed to form autonomous groups. Figures 3.6 and 3.7 are simple flowcharts showing the main features of the 'production flows' through the in-patient and outpatient units.

Later, we shall discuss these matters in relation to the hospital's resources, its participants, its organisation, and 'production conditions'. For the time being, our intention is to present an introductory picture of the hospital in terms that are as simple as possible. Everything reported thus far was part of the picture that we had when our more systematic study and analysis of the hospital was begun.

29

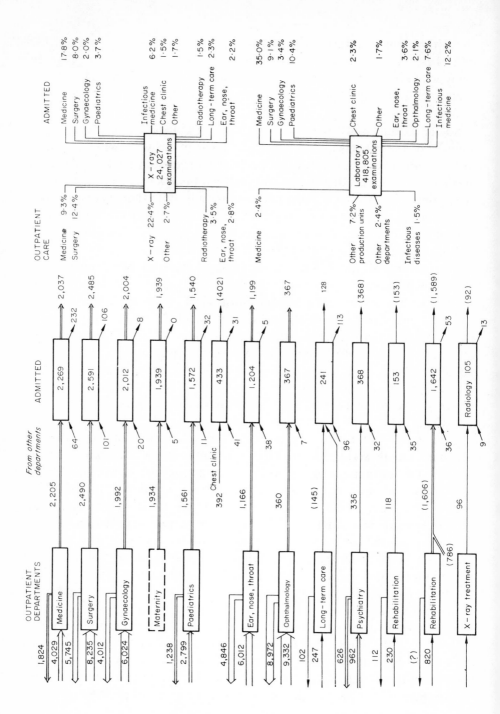

Fig. 3.5 Patient flows at General Hospital.[7]

30

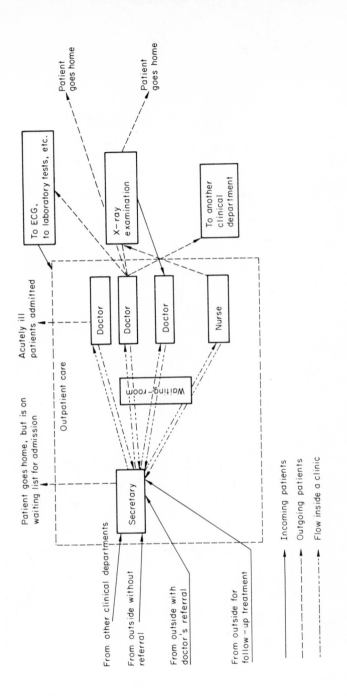

Fig. 3.6   Patient's routes (production flows) in the outpatient clinics.

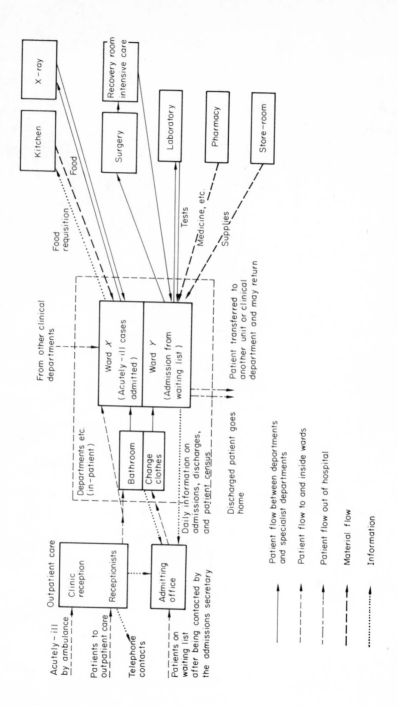

Fig. 3.7   Patients' routes (production flows)—in-patient care.

32

Attitudes in the hospital towards the study

From what we could gather on the basis of these preliminary interviews our introduction to the hospital was successful in that we were generally well-received. Throughout the study we usually found a positive attitude in the hospital towards our presence and the study we were carrying out. The following summaries and excerpts from our earliest notes give some idea of how we think the hospital staff felt about us and our research:

After our description of the research project a department chief said: 'It's a good thing you'll finally be able to show that there are differences between a hospital and industry.'

Many doctors who had worked since early morning are anxious to reserve some time in the evening to stay and talk to us. We are often welcome to visit them during coffee breaks to discuss various problems. The doctors say they are willing to participate in an evening discussion over a glass of beer.

One surgeon is very interested in our research and even offered to participate in the research group. (He later received a short leave of absence for this purpose. This was extremely valuable to us, particularly for his help with medical terminology).

One of the supervisory nurses expressed her hopes about our research as follows: 'The chief nurse has always been underpaid. The hospital is a man's world. You researchers can put that in your report.'

Several people offered to help us collect data. One department chief offered to gather data from doctors in private practice in town. (The fact that he forgot to do so, despite several reminders, perhaps decreased the value of his offer but his intentions were good.)

As could be expected, we also met with some scepticism. This was caused to some extent by our own inability to specify what we would actually be doing. One of the purposes of our pilot study was, in fact, to identify variables to be described.

Dr A put off meeting us for about three or four weeks. (This is probably the same strategy that doctors are forced to apply to troublesome patients who seek them unnecessarily.)

There was a great deal of confusion when we sat down among the doctors in the lunch room. When it was discovered that we were not new or substitute doctors, comments were: 'Are you here to rationalise us?' before they disappeared to the coffee lounge with their cups.

The only time Dr B could see us was either on Walpurgis Eve (April 30) or May Day (both national holidays in Sweden). This doctor was on call then and our interpretation was that either he didn't want to talk to us or that he was anxious to show us how inconvenient his hours were.

The charge nurses were very interested in our talk today. But some of them seemed slightly confused by our behaviour. Nurse C expressed her feelings as follows: 'There are so many people running around interviewing us, observing us and writing down what we do. Why do you always choose my unit?' (It should be noted that this nurse had previously been subjected to time and motion studies performed by experts from a central public health agency, observed by the county council's organisation expert, and interviewed by the consulting firm that was investigating personnel conditions when our study was in progress.)

Other earlier studies of the hospital helped us in the sense that some of the personnel had been in contact with 'investigators' and accepted the fact that we were simply 'a continuation'. Thus, we were accepted even if people were dubious as to what we really had in mind. It should be noted, however, that the other studies were also an obstacle in the sense that we were easily identified with the consultants who studied the personnel situation and gave advice about the functions of the personnel department in the hospital. Many persons also told us their views as to what they thought should be changed—from the lifts, which were always out of order, to unfair treatment of the older nurses.

The current hospital debate seemed to create mixed feelings among the personnel.

Naturally we're very much bound by routine. I certainly don't believe in these changes but you can't say so without being labelled reactionary. Why is everyone talking about so-called opposition to rationalisation? We've always rationalised at hospitals and always will. We need incentives from all directions imaginable.

Assurances that our job was not to propose concrete changes in the hospital or to make time and motion studies usually had a calming effect. The

34

general attitude towards outsider's suggestions for concrete improvements was one of scepticism.

Outsiders don't understand. This isn't industry. You have to have experience from hospitals. We always admitted—quite honestly—that we felt these were highly justifiable views.

Our declaration that we were primarily interested in comparing the hospital with other types of organisations in order to emphasise differences and similarities was also perceived as something positive.

External environment of the hospital

The hospital is located in a typical Swedish industrial town. At the beginning of the nineteenth century when the hospital was founded, the population of Industry Town was about 1,800. This figure grew to approximately 3,500 by 1850. Three industries came to the town during the first half of the twentieth century. These companies, which have grown and still dominate the town, manufacture diesel engines, tractors, household products, measuring instruments, etc. There are also a number of small engineering firms. The number of inhabitants is now around 60,000.

The county council and its offices are located in another city (see Fig. 3.8), even though General Hospital is the largest hospital in the county's jurisdiction. There are three other hospitals in the county.[8] A certain amount of competition for county funds is apparent with respect to obtaining new resources. There are about twenty doctors in private practice in the town, and seven district medical officers who have good contacts with the hospital and use many of its service units, e.g. X-ray and the central laboratory. They also refer patients to the hospital.

Conclusions

Our first impressions of the hospital supported the general opinions expressed earlier by our advisers at the central health agencies. The hospital seemed 'easily accessible' with respect to location and the attitudes of the people working there. We even felt welcome in many instances. The hospital appeared to be 'normal' in terms of size, resources, orientation of activities, and environment. Nothing we observed indicated that the hospital was anything but 'well-run', with the staff working intensively at all levels.

35

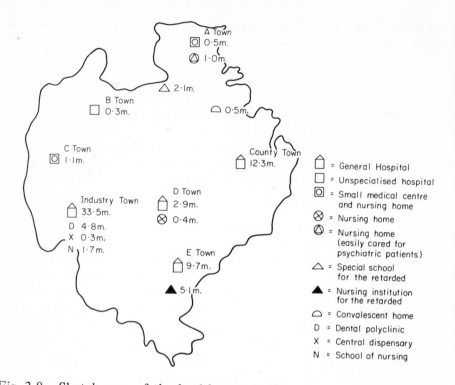

Fig. 3.8 Sketch map of the health care facilities in the county.* (Numbers refer to operating costs in millions of crowns.)

* There are also twenty-three district medical officers in the county. Their operating costs amounted to 0.7 million cr. in 1965. There are nineteen maternity and paediatric clinics located at General Hospital in Industry Town, at the hospitals in County Council Town, C Town, D Town, and E Town. Total operating costs for all these clinics were 0.7 million cr. in 1965. The operating costs for rural public health and medical care (administered primarily by public health nurses) amounted to 2 million cr. in 1965.

Notes

[1] The distinction between city and county hospitals in the Stockholm area was eliminated on 1 January 1971. All these hospitals now belong to the Stockholm County Council.

[2] Burling, T., Lentz, E. M. and Wilson, R. M. (eds.), *The Give and Take*

36

in Hospitals—A Study of Human Organisation, New York 1965.

[3] Dunham, H. W. and Weinberg, S. K., *The Culture of the State Mental Hospital*, Detroit 1960, p. 14.

[4] Ibid, p. 268.

[5] With respect to the most highly specialised types of medical care, Sweden is divided into seven regions, each of which has its own regional hospital.

[6] Unless otherwise stated, the information reported in this and subsequent chapters refers to General Hospital in 1965.

[7] Figure 3.5 shows the patient flow at the hospital. The figures indicating the number of patients and percentages are based on the hospital's statistics. Some of the sources of error are as follows: an acutely-ill person admitted via the outpatient clinic is generally not registered. In other words, a flowchart such as this could not be constructed if many of those admitted to the hospital were not originally outpatients who were put on the waiting list for admission. In addition, most of the outpatients treated probably made at least one follow-up visit to the outpatient clinic. This applies even if the patient is referred from another hospital in the county.

The X-ray department performed work for other institutions. Use of these services was debited by the same method used in distributing the X-ray department's costs. This means that service requested from other clinical departments was graded according to norms formulated by the Association of County Councils. The central laboratory's services were distributed in accordance with the number of tests performed for the different specialties during two periods (3-15 March and 1-15 October 1964).

[8] There are also three mental hospitals in the county. A large number of patients from outside the county are hospitalised at two of them. These hospitals were state-owned until 1 January 1967, after which they became the property of the county council.

37

4 The Hospital's Participant Relations

A major tenet of organisation theory is that the internal functioning of an organisation, including its administration, depends a great deal on the environment in which it operates. The participants comprise the most important part of the environment. Here the term 'participants' refers to the individuals or groups that directly depend on the organisation to realise their own personal goals and on whom the organisation depends to attain its own objectives. Customers, owners, employees, suppliers, lenders, state and local government are examples of some important participants in industrial firms. The hospital's participants will be studied in this chapter.

Selection of the relationships for study was guided primarily by our expectations as to the most important relations between the hospital's participants and its production (see Fig. 4.1). We investigated the participants contributions to production at the hospital, and the inducements they received in return. This enabled us to become acquainted with some of the most significant factors affecting the hospital's production, especially as the requirements placed on the hospital's products subsequently affect the production system and production control. The description of the institutions used by the hospital to resolve conflicts with participants, and the analysis of the participants' relative power and internal relations were motivated primarily by the importance of the demands that these factors place on the hospital's participant administration.

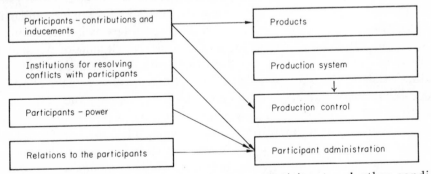

Fig. 4.1 Some important relations between participant and other conditions at the hospital.

39

Defining the range of the hospital

When we refer to the strategy of the hospital we mean the set of participants chosen by the hospital, and the institutions used by the hospital to establish working relations with these participants in order to resolve potential conflicts. But before its strategy can be studied, the hospital has to be defined and its range and boundaries set. There are units on the hospital grounds, and even inside the hospital itself, which are not formally parts of the hospital (see Table 4.1).[1] The chest X-ray unit, dental clinic, and county orthodontist are all directly under the county council but are located in buildings which otherwise belong to the hospital. The School of Nursing, a training school for nurses' aides, and the central laundry are all located in separate buildings on the hospital grounds. The pharmacy is a branch of a pharmacy in town, though it functions as the hospital's own unit. A subsidiary of the county council's central purchasing agency is next to the orthopaedic outpatient clinic. This unit produces and tests orthopaedic braces and appliances for use throughout Sweden.

For this study, we have defined the range and boundaries of the hospital on the basis of its formal structure. Only the units formally under the hospital's administration (see Fig. 3.4) were classified as belonging to the hospital, regardless of the real influence exerted by the hospital's board of directors, the director of the hospital, or the department chiefs on these units.

The hospital's participants—introductory survey

To begin with, we tried to identify the participants and classify them into groups giving more or less similar contributions and receiving similar inducements. Our method has primarily involved interviewing those of the staff who could be expected to have a good overall view of participant relations (see Fig. 4.2). On the basis of the hospital's annual report and other available documents, we made a preliminary survey of the contribution-inducement balance, i.e. the contributions made by the participants and the inducements they receive in return (Table 4.2).[2] (A brief account of the participants we identified is also included.) Incentives refer to extra inducements given to the participants to encourage increased contributions. The main flows of contributions and inducements are shown in Figure 4.3.

On the basis of this introductory survey, we made the following obser-

40

TABLE 4.1

Components outside the formal boundaries of the hospital.[3]

Components not formally part of the hospital	Most important points of contact with the hospital
Central county dental clinic (including dental surgery)	Located within the hospital. The ear, nose, and throat department often refers patients to this component
County orthodontic clinic	Located within the hospital. Few contacts with the hospital itself.
Spastic care unit	Located within the hospital. Certain personnel in common.
Maternity centre	Located within the hospital. Some personnel in common with the obstetrics and gynaecology departments. Most of the patients are taken over by obstetrics and gynaecology.
Polio and scarlet fever unit	Meets at the hospital once a month. Staffed by personnel from the hospital.
One of the county's chest X-ray units	Facilities at the hospital. Some personnel from the chest clinic. Patients requiring hospitalisation are taken care of by the chest clinic.
Local training school for nursing auxiliaries	Facilities and training at the hospital.
County School of Nursing	Facilities on the hospital grounds. Students and teachers eat in the hospital dining-room. Training at the hospital. Participation in writing nursing policy and procedure book. Some administration in common.
County purchasing agency, prosthesis workshop	Located within the hospital. Referral of patients from the department of orthopaedics. Close cooperation with physicians.
Child health centre	Located within the hospital. Some personnel from the department of paediatrics. Some patients referred to the department of paediatrics.

vations. Only a very limited amount of the services provided by the hospital are paid for directly by the patients (see Fig. 4.3). Payments in the outpatient clinics are made to the doctors, who then repay a certain sum per patient and visit to the hospital (1.60 cr. in 1965).[4] Costs for X-ray film are paid to the hospital. The county authorities are responsible for

41

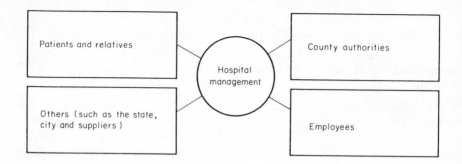

Fig. 4.2   General Hospital's most important participants.

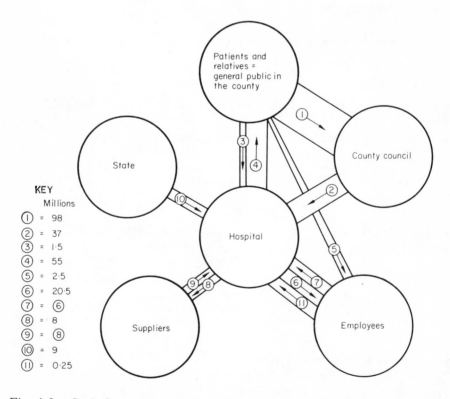

Fig. 4.3   Cash flows (in crowns) between General Hospital and its participants

42

providing most of the hospital's economic resources. General Hospital is an important part of their budget. Most of the money from this source goes to wages and salaries. If the exchange of goods and services is added to the cash flows, we find a two-way flow between the hospital and its employees and the hospital and its suppliers. The services rendered by the hospital to the public, the taxes paid by the public, and the county's allocations to the hospital form a kind of triangle. This in turn influences individual incentives in that none of the three groups included in the triangle receives any extra inducement if it makes extra contributions.

Participant power and the institutions for resolving conflicts

Most organisations have difficulty in satisfying the demands of their participants, at least in the long run. This is the result of a general scarcity of need fulfilment in society; also, the fact that the participants' demands are often contradictory. Cooperation between the various parties concerned thus becomes part of the overall strategy and affects the participants' chances of having their demands met by the organisation.

Our impressions of the institutions set up by General Hospital for resolving conflicts were based on interviews with people at the hospital who are in contact with the various participants. Supplementary interviews with representatives of the participants were made in some cases.

We also tried to estimate the power of the different participants, i.e. their opportunities to use sanctions or other means to assert their demands and see that they are met. But theories in this area are poorly developed and our analysis is inconclusive and unsystematic. A survey of these institutions is shown in Table 4.3. More detailed comments are included for some of the most important participants.

The most characteristic feature of the institutions that the hospital uses to resolve conflicts and promote cooperation with its participants is that—as opposed to the situation in a large industrial firm—only a few of them can be described in market terms. Instead, consultation and negotiation are used to a large extent. But sometimes the participants have direct influence over the decision-making process at the hospital, most notably the county authorities (the formal owner of the hospital), i.e. the county council. The hospital depends on the county authorities much more than a large company depends on its stockholders. Through a unilateral decision the county authorities can shut down General Hospital. This could happen, for example, if they decided to combine all medical units in the county into a hospital in another town. The hospital's dependence on the

43

TABLE 4.2

Contribution-inducement balance at General Hospital

Contributions	Inducements	Incentives
County authorities COUNTY COUNCIL (political) Approves appropriations to the hospital. Operating budget 1965: 27.9 million cr. Capital budget 1960-65, average 0.99 million cr./year.	*Preparedness* (ability to provide service) No. of beds per 10,000 inhabitants in the hospital district. Average no. of beds at General Hospital.	
COUNTY COUNCIL OFFICE STAFF (full-time salaried) Contributes some resources for special studies.		
Hospitalised patients Pay hospitalisation fees (via national social insurance). See County Council. Approx. 1.5 million cr.	*Care* Mean no. of beds occupied per day: 641.9. No. of patient days: 234,000 costing at least 107 cr./day. No. of patients: 15,800 costing at least 1,590 cr./patient.	Semi-private room for 15 cr./day. Private room for 30 cr./day[5]

44

Average length of stay: 10.4 days (excluding chronic care, psychiatry and chest clinics).

Additional contribution not formally permitted (if the patient is admitted to the hospital his financial contribution is considerably reduced).

Outpatient care
Pay doctor fees according to a fixed rate (approx. 7-30 cr./visit) 75%[6] of which is refunded by the national insurance service.
Lost working time: approx. 2.5 million cr.

Examination and treatment
Outpatient visits/consultations (excluding X-ray examinations): 116,000.
No. of patients: 48,000.

For in-patient care: usually 40 cr./bed and year.
For outpatient care: usually 50-250 cr./hour.

Personnel
DEPARTMENT CHIEFS (16)
Working time:[7] approx. 50 hours/week. Not directly on call but serve as back-up during alternate 24-hour periods.

SALARY LEVEL KB1[8]
Some department chiefs receive compensation/bed for in-patient care: 40 cr. (maternity beds, 20 cr.).
Department chiefs with limited in-patient care: up to 18,000 cr. extra/year.
Pathologists: compensation for each test, and an additional 1,200 cr./year.
Other department chiefs:
Psychiatrists, 5,500 cr.

45

Contributions	Inducements	Incentives
	Specialists in child psychiatry, 18,000 cr. Specialists in infectious diseases, 7,500 cr. Rehabilitation, 10,000 cr. Total income from work: approx. 1.15 million cr.	
OTHER DOCTORS (40) Working time: 45-60 hours/week (no fixed working hours). On call up to 80 hours/week.	SALARY LEVEL KA 22 (Deputy department chief A25) Permission for junior doctor to receive patients for outpatient treatment. Compensation with time off corresponding to time on call or 11 cr./hour. Total income from work: approx. 1.54 million cr.	For in-patient care: nothing. For outpatient care: 50-250 cr./hour.[9] Care contribution not decisive factor for promotion.
NURSING PERSONNEL (850) Working time: 42.5 hours/week, including Sundays and holidays; otherwise 45 hours/week.	SALARY LEVELS Registered nurses, KA 13-15. Assistant nurses, KA 10-12. Nursing auxiliaries, KA 3-7. Total income approx. 12.78 million cr.	On-call compensation: 1.50-3 cr./hour (i.e. approx. 200 cr. extra/month for most nurses). Compensation for inconvenient working hours: 1.42 cr./hour.

MAINTENANCE PERSONNEL (100) Working time: 45 hours/week	SALARY LEVEL KA 3-7 (10) Total income from work: approx. 2.06 million cr.	Compensation for overtime.
ADMINISTRATIVE AND OTHER PERSONNEL (32) Working time: 42 hours/week	SALARY LEVELS Director's assistant, KA 23. Special studies secretary, KA21. Personnel assistant, KA 17-19. Hospital assistant, KA 17. Chief nurse, KA 21. Supervisory nurse, KA 16. Comptroller, KA 21. Personnel chief, KA 23. Total income from work: approx. 0.66 million cr.	Increased possibilities for promotion
HOSPITAL MANAGEMENT Hospital director, working time: 50 hours/week Chief of the medical staff, part-time (18 hours/week). Members of the hospital board: 14 regular meetings (1-2 hours each) and at least 12 subcommittee meetings (4-5 hours each).	SALARY LEVELS Hospital director, KB1. Remuneration Chief of the medical staff, 10,000 cr. Chairman, 5,000 cr. Board members, 50-65 cr./meeting. Total compensation from the hospital approx. 75,000 cr.	No economic incentives.

47

Contributions	Inducements	Incentives
Other participants		
STATE		
Contributes 1.50-3 cr./day to certain departments (chronic care, infectious medicine, psychiatry, child psychiatry, paediatrics and chest clinics) for constructing and equipping of facilities. Various central agencies (National Board of Health, Central Board of Hospitals Planning, National Council for Hospital Rationalisation)[10] Total state subsidy: approx. 151,000 cr.	Possibility of controlling the hospital to some extent.	
INDUSTRY TOWN		
Supplies water and electricity to the hospital. Has offered five home sites for sale to hospital personnel.	In providing employment for the female labour force, General Hospital increases the status of the town.	Larger tax base to make it easier for better-paid personnel to reside in the district.

The hospital takes some of the strain from the district nursing home.

Taxes from employees at the hospital: approx. 5 million cr.

Assured payment of approx. 6.5 million cr. but often with a high discount.

SUPPLIERS
Goods

county authorities is similar to that of a subsidiary or local branch's dependence on the parent company. The hospital can be regarded as an appendix organisation to the county council.[11]

The hospital can use the market as the most important institution for resolving conflicts in relation only to its suppliers and personnel. But stable cooperation has not been established with these two participants to the same extent as in most large industrial firms. An exception to this is the pharmacy in Industry Town which is a permanent supplier since it has been allowed to set up a branch at the hospital. Of course, through the county authorities, the hospital is a partner in the county council's central purchasing agency and is thus expected to make certain purchases there. But with few exceptions the hospital has retained the right to make most purchases freely.

Certain participants usually make payments direct to one another. The most important examples are the taxes paid by the general public to the county authorities and the patients' fees to physicians. These payments are regulated through institutions for resolving conflicts which are wholly beyond the control of the hospital management. Taxes are set through the democratic decision-making process in the county council. Patient fees in the outpatient clinics (hospital-doctor fees) are determined through negotiations between the Association of County Councils and the Swedish Medical Association.[12] So in this case, the hospital does not assume the task of resolving conflicts. This coincides with the current trend in Sweden whereby most firms transfer their wage setting to collective bargaining between the central employer and employee organisations. There is also another more limited, but perhaps more significant example of the hospital management's passive role in bargaining. While our study was in progress there were several instances of direct negotiations between the department chiefs and junior doctors, with—and even without—the participation of the hospital management. These negotiations were aimed at settling matters (such as the on-call system) affecting the interests of these two employee groups. Direct negotiations were also carried out between junior doctors in two departments as to the conditions for cooperation between these two departments.

There is a similar triangular relation between the hospital, the National Board of Health and Welfare, and various licensed personnel (doctors, nurses, physiotherapists, and midwives). The National Board has to maintain certain standards of care and treatment. This is accomplished primarily through sanctions which can be imposed on licensed personnel. These sanctions include a reminder, a warning, revoking of authorisation to practise a profession or activity under the auspices of the board, and

50

TABLE 4.3

The hospital's most important institutions for resolving conflicts

Participant	Institution for resolving conflicts	Participant's most important means of exerting power	The hospital's most important means of exerting power
County authorities	Augment the board (direct influence on the decision making process at the hospital).	Refuse to approve appropriations or to make other decisions (e.g. about new positions).	Transfer responsibility for unsatisfactory medical care to county authorities
Patients	Complaint procedure.	Convey complaints to next level. Write to newspapers.	Patient's idea of the hospital's power is very unclear. Perhaps the patient thinks that if he complains he will receive inferior care the next time he becomes ill.
Personnel			
Department chiefs	Participation in board Meetings	Professional authority: I cannot be held medically accountable for the consequences	
Other employees	Job market. Collective bargaining.	Quit their jobs. Picket. Strike (to a limited extent).	Decisions as to promotion, Assigning sought-after tasks. Blacklisting. Lock-out
Other participants			
The state	Augment the board. Licensing. Inspection.	Revoke subsidies. Ration job appointments for doctors. Invoke sanctions against licensed personnel.	Transfer responsibility for unsatisfactory medical care to the state
The city	Personal cooperation	Refuse to allot housing (controls land required for expanding the hospital).	
Suppliers	Market.	Refuse to deliver.	Refuse to buy.

finally, legal action. [13] The head of the hospital division of the National Board of Health and Welfare sometimes conducts inspections. General Hospital has not, however, been visited for several years.

Power of individual participants

The county council

The organisation of the county council should be explained to show how it influences General Hospital. Figure 4.4 is a simplified organisation chart. The county council is a politically elected body which usually meets one week in every year. The executive committee with its full-time chairman is the working body directly under the county council. Half the fourteen members of the committee constitute the health and medical services board, the other seven, the finance department. Members of the committee form other permanent or temporary agencies such as the building committee, the wages board, and the rationalisation committee. The administrative staff of the county council has been enlarged considerably during the past few years, and now has about forty employees. The office is headed by a county director who supervises different departments and sections. Organisation of the administration was being revised while our study was in progress.

The most important task of the county council is to determine a budget, which includes provision for health and medical care. The hospital laws and code stipulate the following with respect to the health and medical services board:

> According to this law, health and medical service activities of the county council district are controlled by the type of board referred to in section 53 of the County Council Act, designated the Health and Medical Services Board.
>
> The Health and Medical Services Board has to be attentive to the requirements and development of medical care and make proposals to the county or city council. The Board should promote as much planned development of medical care as possible.[14]

It is the duty of the Board:

1 to prescribe reports and proposals on measures in the area of public health and medical care for the county council or city council to decide on;

52

2 to make proposals for the division of the public health area into medical districts;

3 when required, to propose changes in basic hospital fees;

4 to propose required expansion and changes at the hospital, and, on approval by the county or city council to undertake constructional

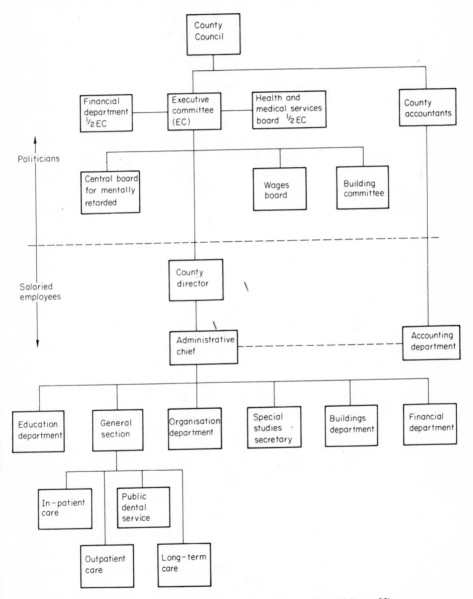

Fig. 4.4 Organisation chart of the county council and its offices.

work, extensions and structural changes which are of such magnitude that they cannot be included in ordinary maintenance;

5 in reference to districts with several district medical officers, to allocate medical care tasks among them;

6 to determine at which hospitals, departments, and other facilities outpatient care should be administered, to the extent that the county and city council does not decide such matters;

7 to the extent it finds suitable, and with county or city council approval to arrange for common purchasing, heating, laundry or other activities covering several hospitals;

8 to present the hospitals' Boards of Trustees with directives, reminders, and instructions with reference to the hospitals' administration;

9 according to directives of the National Board of Health and Welfare, to present before the end of March, a report covering activities in the various medical districts during the year prior to the preceding calendar year, and covering activities at hospitals (including information on the number of beds and patients as well as a financial report) before the end of April; and

10 to otherwise carry out the duties of the Health and Medical Services Board in accordance with requirements and decisions made by the county or city council.

In order to promote planned development in public health and medical care, the Health and Medical Services Board should, after consultation with the authorities in question, draft plans for different areas of public health and medical care.[15]

The county council's influence on the hospital is primarily derived from its task of determining operating, investment, and personnel budgets. As in most areas of public administration, budget reviews usually concentrate on increases in relation to the preceding year's budget. Despite this emphasis, there are unlimited possibilities for controlling everything related to changes in conditions at the hospital. Interviews with leading members of the county council and its staff indicate awareness of the need to delegate matters to local agencies, but in practice, the council still exerts considerable control in all significant areas. This is well illustrated in Table 4.4 which shows the most important matters which the hospital's board of trustees referred to the health and medical services board or other agencies in the county council for decision.

Fairly recently, General Hospital wanted to convert some shower

54

facilities into a dining-room (cost 17,000 cr.). This matter had to be formally approved by the county council even though the hospital director had to consult the county council building committee about implementing this kind of change. When a department chief wants to take a day's leave of absence with pay to attend a conference, the executive committee's wages board has to give its approval. When the hospital wanted to revise its store-room accounting system, the executive committee had to authorise the change (because a 13,700 cr. appropriation was required).

The real influence exerted by the county council over certain decisions at the hospital depends to a large extent on the financial resources which it controls for support of such items, and to a lesser extent, on the personal ambitions of the leading council members and its full-time staff. The county council and its personnel are—probably rightly—convinced that they have better resources for special studies than General Hospital and that they are thus in a better position to make evaluations. One

TABLE 4.4

Matters referred by the hospital's board of trustees to the county council, or its agencies, for decision

Decision	Controlling agency	Approximate no. of decisions per year
Changes in salary-grades	Executive committee	2-3
Requests for extra funds, i.e. for expenses not included in the ordinary budget	Executive committee	5-6
Changes in use of facilities	Health and medical services board [16]	2-3
Entertainment and courtesies	Executive commitee	3-4
Revenue and expenditure estimates	County council	1
Proposals for new specialties or other new or expanded activities at the hospital	Health and medical services board	1-2
Rationalisation or organisation studies requiring extra funds	Health and medical services board	2-3
Reallocation of appropriated funds	Health and medical services board	1-2
Establishment of and changes in medical appointments	National Board of Health and Welfare	3

Table 4.4 (continued)

Establishment of and changes in other positions	County council	50
Appointment and dismissal of department chiefs	County council and Swedish government	1-2
Appointment and dismissal of hospital director, chief of medical staff, deputy department chiefs and junior physicians	Health and medical services board	10-15
Appointment of locum doctors, nurses and physiotherapists without Swedish licenses	National Board of Health and Welfare	30
Scrutiny of health certificates for pensions	Wages board	5-10
Permission to do spare-time work	Health and medical services board	Seldom
Scrutiny of wage and employment conditions for the partially disabled	Wages board	Seldom
Scrutiny, in some cases, of credit from previous employment for salary placement	Wages board	25-30
Scrutiny of fringe benefits during leaves of absence in cases other than illness, pregnancy, military service, refresher courses, conferences, etc.	Wages board	75-100
Compiling list of positions which include housing accommodations	Wages board	Seldom
Setting rent for housing accommodations	Housing board	Seldom
Setting prices in personnel dining room	Executive committee	Every third year
Pensions	Government employee pensions board, executive committee	10-15
Group life insurance	Public insurance company	Seldom
Periodical travel allowances, home-job site	Wages board	25-30

56

influential employee put the council's position as follows: 'From now on, no new personnel appointments will be approved until we have made an organisation study.' But one leading politician implied that the hospital's board of trustees would probably increase its freedom of action because it had improved its own staff resources.

This central control is partly due to the fact that the county council itself is controlled. For instance, when General Hospital wanted to convert a psychiatric ward into an orthopaedic ward, the county council executive committee had to submit a request to the Swedish Government because the State had once granted a subsidy amounting to 15 per cent of the initial cost. This request has to be repeated annually since this approval is valid for only a year at a time. The wages board's careful scrutiny of even rather small matters is understandable, since it, in turn, is checked by the county council's accountants.

The patients

The hospital's board of trustees is appointed by the county council, and its membership more or less reflects the council's political party structure. Thus, the first way in which patients can make their demands known at the hospital is through their democratic voting rights. This gives the voters an opportunity to voice their disapproval of an administration which does not protect their interests. The same applies to the county council and its different agencies, i.e. the executive committee and the health and medical services board. We interviewed some trustees, council members, and journalists with good access to political authorities, to find out how the political decision-making process functions in respect to health care.

Health and medical care is not an issue that adheres to party lines. There has hardly been any public discussion in which the various parties have advocated different programmes in this area. However, in the 1966 elections the Liberal and Conservative opposition did include local health issues in their overall criticism of 'the queueing society'. In local election debates and the local press, the opposition claimed that the Social Democrats had waited too long to deal with the education of medical personnel and had neglected housing problems. On several occasions, the Conservative Party has demanded lower tax levies, provided that the plans agreed by all parties could still be financed. Bills proposed by various parties have demanded an increase in resources allocated to different groups in need of medical care.

Some of the hospital's trustees and county members felt that the

57

various parties are wary of each other, and that all of them are extremely afraid to seem unambitious or uninterested in health care issues. Immediately before the county council election in 1966, we interviewed some leading Social Democrats who emphasised that they thought the amount of time spent in outpatient waiting-rooms was an important political problem. They felt pressure from the voters. The same problem had been mentioned six months earlier, but in a less pronounced manner. Of course, new facilities and increased medical services have to be weighed against limitations on tax increases. Limited resources always imply that priority has to be given to certain needs. Health care issues handled by the county council compete with other needs such as vocational training. In addition, most party groups think that there is competition between county and municipal interests. The municipalities have various needs, and an increase in county taxes usually limits the chance to increase city taxes. The politicial authorities function primarily as an institution for determining the amount of resources that will be spent on health and medical care. This is directly related to resolving the conflict between medical interests and other public needs and between public needs as a whole and demands for private consumption and saving. Thus, comparisons between tax levels and county taxes in other counties receive a great deal of attention: 'The county tax is 6 cr. per 100 cr. here, and the national average is 5.95 cr. per 100 cr. so a general increase is not politically feasible' (according to several of our interviewees).[17]

The most politically sensitive issues handled by the county council, i.e. those which tend to be most controversial, are construction of small medical centres, and the standards set there. In this instance, the differences in opinion traverse party lines, and the conflict is mostly between local interests and those of the public at large. The democratic decision-making process functions as it should in this area, with intensive public discussions in the press, letters-to-the editor, disagreements within the parties and the county council, as well as political sanctions (i.e. no re-election) of representatives who do not protect the expressed interests of the voters, e.g. when common interests are given priority over local interests. But these issues have not affected General Hospital to a large extent, and some of the interviewees described them as 'old-fashioned petty politics'.

If a patient group is sufficiently large and well organised, it might be given special attention by some ambitious politician and may even be able to negotiate directly with the decision-making health authorities. For instance, patient organisations can carry on campaigns in the press, send out delegations, and present their demands as bills put before the county

58

council through individual representatives. Later, we shall show that these opportunities have only been used to a limited extent.

The patient regards the hospital as an institution with an almost absolute monopoly position. Patients in Industry Town who require hospitalisation seldom go to private hospitals. There are private hospitals a few hours away in Big City, but inquiries to department chiefs and private nursing homes in Big City provided us with only a few, isolated cases of patients taking advantage of this opportunity. Of course, this is the result of the high cost of treatment and care at private institutions. The outpatient units at the hospital do 'compete' with doctors in private practice, as well as with city and district physicians. But these groups cannot usually provide the same level of care as the hospital. Thus far, there are no group practices in Industry Town. So the patients' most effective method of making themselves heard is to complain. Complaints are dealt with as follows: first, within a department where the department chief is the highest decision-making authority; second, outside the clinical department where there are different procedures depending on the nature of the complaint.

The hospital management

Our investigation of the power of the hospital's management does not include its overall influence in the hospital, but is directed at its potential for realising its own demands for inducements (mainly salaries). It turns out that the hospital director, chief of the medical staff, and members of the board all belong to different unions. The hospital director belongs to the Swedish Confederation of Professional Associations. He is not assigned to a salary level in accordance with the lists agreed through collective bargaining. But the hospital director's chances of receiving a higher salary depend to a large extent on how well hospital directors as a group can protect their interests, since the various county councils watch each other carefully in these matters. The same principle applies to the medical staff, department chiefs, and members of the hospital's board, though these groups receive different fringe benefits in different hospitals and counties. The last time that the salaries of the chief of the medical staff and the board of trustees were raised, the county council made all decisions as to levels and fringe benefits.

59

The department chiefs

The department chiefs rely primarily on two organisations for asserting their demands: the Swedish Association of Hospital Doctors and General Hospital's department chiefs' association. The former is a national professional organisation with two representatives in the county. The Association negotiates with the Swedish Association of County Councils via the Swedish Medical Association. The local representatives seldom serve as negotiators.[18]

The department chiefs' association is an informal institution. Meetings are called at the discretion of the chairman to discuss issues of mutual interest, such as new methods for examining patients, library matters, and assorted administrative problems. The group met eight times in 1965, and these meetings lasted between two and five hours. 'Nearly all' the department chiefs participated. The association also serves as an advisory body to the board of trustees in regard to legislative proposals. But the group is not very effective as a pressure group within the hospital, because there are often differences of opinion on important issues, and some statements said to represent the association as a whole do not have the support of all members. The chief of the medical staff, who participates in board meetings and is a member of the executive committee, does not try to use the association as a means of exerting pressure on the trustees. Instead, the association serves as an instrument for consultation, and to some extent, for resolving differences of opinion among the department chiefs. One of the associations' duties was to propose how a 25,000 cr. research grant from the county council should be distributed among doctors in the county. The department chiefs and hospital's management deny that one, or several, of the department chiefs have a dominating influence on their colleagues. [19] We have made no observations to the contrary.

One doctor described the department chiefs' association as follows:

> The department chiefs influence each other somewhat with regard to requests for grants in the sense that certain requests are opposed, while other chiefs are encouraged to request funds for certain equipment. One department chief who wanted a new position for a junior doctor was opposed by other chiefs who felt he had gone too far. But obviously, if a department chief is highly interested in something he somehow gets it accomplished. For instance, Dr A recently acquired new equipment costing 120,000 cr. while the real need for this equipment was debatable from the hospital's point of view. The department chiefs' association has probably been formed to protect

60

the interests of the chiefs from politicians and administrative suppression. This kind of cooperation is probably necessary. When I worked at another hospital there was a case where the X-ray department requested a certain apparatus. The hospital director went to the head of surgery and asked him if he would have any use for it. In other words, the director pitted the two department chiefs against each other, and the whole thing was very unpleasant. This is one example that illustrates why the department chiefs discovered they had to cooperate to some extent. But things like this hardly ever happen in Industry Town so the group is not so necessary here.

The chief of the medical staff participates in board of trustee meetings and is included in its executive subcommittee. The department chiefs' demands should formally be made to the hospital through the chief of the medical staff and the trustees. However, the individual department chief often prefers to contact the chief of the medical staff when he has some demand to make. But this route is not always a matter of course. If a department chief thinks he can gain more by other routes he uses them, regardless of whether this involves direct contact with the chairman of the board, employees and members of the county council, or the National Board of Health and Welfare. The department chiefs often take part in board meetings. They may participate in discussions pertaining to their own clinical departments (but not in decisions). The relatively limited importance of the department chiefs' association probably stems from the fact that an organisation for protecting common interests is not really necessary. The individual department chief has sufficiently strong means at his disposal to realise his demands. His most important asset is his professional knowledge. When a department chief says that 'he will not assume medical responsibility for the consequences ...', there are not many laymen who dare to contradict him.[20] This professional authority can also be used for more far-reaching measures. A department chief can make public statements about conditions that he feels are unsatisfactory. But these, and similar measures, can only be used with certain types of demands—particularly those for increased resources. They are not usually helpful to the department chief who wants to acquire personal advantages, even though increased resources for the hospital are often accompanied by advantages to the department chiefs as a group. The hospital has no 'countermeasures' for dealing with the department chiefs' strong position. A department chief possesses a 'royal letter' which means that he cannot be dismissed unless he commits a criminal act. This, combined with the department chiefs' salary system, means that the hospital lacks three of

61

the most important means of influencing employee behaviour that are used in industrial firms: control of promotions, hiring and firing, and determination of salaries. The hospital board does have certain means at its disposal through budget control and allocation of resources, but these are counteracted by very strong pressure from the doctors.

Other personnel

Even if we distinguish between the hospital's management and department chiefs (two groups of employees), the participant 'personnel' is still a very heterogeneous group. Power of the personnel applies to the contributions and inducements they exchange with the hospital, general relations between them and the hospital, and their power in relation to the hospital. Our description of the hospital's relations to its personnel contains many important indications of differences between personnel groups.

In analysing the power of the personnel, it might be worthwhile to study the personnel organisations (unions) first. The hospital's employees belong to several unions. The hospital (or rather the central employers' association, the Swedish Association of County Councils), has many collective agreements with the various employee organisations. There are several important differences between these unions in terms of affiliation with different central top employee organisations, orientation towards the hospital as the main employer, size, percentage of organised employees, office resources, strike funds, etc.

The employees' power at General Hospital is only partly—and perhaps not even significantly—based on their organisations. Their bargaining positions depend on either the lack or availability of the services they offer. Statistics on vacancies compiled by the National Board of Health and Welfare illustrate these conditions, and form the basis of Table 4.5. Corresponding data from General Hospital refer to the same period (see Table 4.20); the source is information submitted to the National Board of Health and Welfare by General Hospital. The most noteworthy aspect of the data from General Hospital is the small number of vacancies in the non-licensed groups and the serious lack of assistant nurses, physiotherapists, registered nurses, and doctors.

The situation at General Hospital with regard to doctors and nurses is even more critical than at most somatic hospitals. In reality, the data do not indicate the full seriousness of the situation because many of the positions are filled by substitutes; $126\frac{1}{2}$ of the $202\frac{1}{2}$ nursing jobs are held by permanent staff, 37 by temporary workers, and there are $39\frac{1}{4}$ vacancies (see Table 4.20).

62

TABLE 4.5

Vacancies 1 October 1965

Personnel category	Vacancies (without substitutes) nationwide (%)	Vacancies (without substitutes) at all somatic hospitals (%)	Vacancies (without substitutes) at General Hospital (%)
Doctors	7.6	7.9	12.7
Registered nurses	7.1	8.0	12.6
Midwives	5.2	5.1	0
Physiotherapists	15.6	20.3	35.7
Social workers	10.4	12.9	10.0
Therapists	5.2	5.5	0
Assistant nurses	4.9	2.9	12.2
Paediatric nurses	1.1	2.9	0
Other nursing staff	2.5	1.7	0
Housekeeping staff	3.6	0	0
Office staff	1.1	0	0

Source: National Board of Health and Welfare statistics, Tables 1.1-1.3 and 2.4.

It is interesting to compare vacancy statistics with the different personnel groups' views of their own market position. We tried to measure this by asking the personnel how easy they thought it would be to obtain another job, and how attractive these alternatives were (Tables 4.6 and 4.7).

The average opinion of all personnel as to how easy it is to obtain another job lies between 'it is easy' and 'it is fairly easy' (Table 4.6). These opinions are — quite naturally — influenced by age. Generally, the average opinion of all groups indicates that people over 30 believe that it becomes progressively more difficult to obtain other jobs. But on average, doctors, registered nurses, and other professional categories in particular, think that it would be 'easy to obtain another job' (5.0, 5.0 and 5.2 per cent, respectively). Other nursing, maintenance and office personnel give more

63

cautious evaluations, and the averages for these groups are close to 'fairly easy' (4.3, 4.3, and 4.1 per cent, respectively). The median for other professional categories' and doctors' evaluations is 'it would be very easy to obtain another job'. The median of evaluations by registered nurses is 'it would be easy', while the median for other groups is 'it would be fairly easy'.

Similar results are obtained for the different groups with respect to the age factor. Doctors and registered nurses show higher values than other types of personnel for almost all age groups. The ancillary professional category is represented by so few respondents in most age groups that nothing definite can be said about age variations in this category. Nevertheless, age does seem to affect the evaluation. In general, respondents over 30 think that difficulty in obtaining other jobs increases with age.

The doctors questioned thought it easiest to obtain other jobs in the age groups 21 to 25 and 26 to 30. However, the former age group is somewhat special since it comprises mostly medical students with temporary appointments. The relatively high values for doctors in the 51 to 60 age group can be partly explained by the fact that this group is composed mostly of department chiefs. Registered nurses believe that it is, roughly, equally easy to obtain other jobs in all age groups between 20 and 50, and more difficult thereafter. Other nursing staff think it easiest to obtain other jobs in age groups up to 30. The highest evaluations by maintenance staff are in the lowest age groups (although the number of respondents was too small to yield definite conclusions). As for office staff, the highest evaluations were for age groups 21 to 25 and 31 to 40 (also a very small number of respondents).

In sum, the answers seem to indicate that ancillary professionals, doctors, and registered nurses evaluate their market positions somewhat more favourably than other nursing, maintenance and office staff. There is a high degree of conformity between vacancy statistics and the personnel's own view of available alternative jobs.[21]

The average evaluation of all personnel as to how attractive other jobs are (see Table 4.6) is close to 'they are hardly attractive' (3.2 per cent). The age factor also influences these evaluations in the sense that, after 30, other jobs become less attractive. The averages for different groups show the same tendency as in the job mobility question. The ancillary professional personnel have the highest average value—somewhat above 'fairly attractive' (4.4 per cent) while doctors and nurses gave an average value somewhat below 'fairly attractive' (3.8 per cent). The relatively high average values for ancillary professionals can also be explained in this case by the fact that they are not represented in the two highest age groups.

64

TABLE 4.6

Different employee groups' perception of available alternative jobs

	Doctors (%)	Nurses (%)	Non-professional nursing staff (%)	Other professional staff (%)	Maintenance and other staff (%)	Office staff (%)
Assume that you would like to be employed at some place other than General Hospital. How easy would it be for you to obtain another job?						
(6) It would be very easy	58	44	19	65	16	7
(5) It would be easy	13	25	23	12	26	24
(4) It would be fairly easy	13	22	39	6	36	48
(3) It would be fairly difficult	4	8	14	18	11	10
(2) It would be difficult	6	0	3	0	7	10
(1) It would be very difficult	6	2	2	0	3	0
Mean values	5.0	5.0	4.3	5.2	4.3	4.1
Number of respondents	54	121	277	17	67	31
No answer	1	3	15	0	6	2
How attractive would another job be for you?						
(6) It is very attractive	9	12	4	24	3	3
(5) It is attractive	22	19	6	29	16	10
(4) It is fairly attractive	26	27	15	24	19	27
(3) It is hardly attractive	28	27	33	12	26	33
(2) It is not attractive	6	11	25	6	19	13
(1) It is definitely not attractive	8	5	16	6	16	13
Average values	3.8	3.8	2.8	4.4	3.1	3.2
Number of respondents	54	121	277	17	67	31
No answer	1	9	13	0	5	1

65

TABLE 4.7

Influence of age and job on perception of available jobs

Mean value of answers to the question: How easy would it be for you to obtain another job?

Age group	Personnel group						
	Doctors	Nurses	Non-professional nursing staff	Ancillary professional staff	Maintenance and other staff	Office staff	All personnel
$<$ 21 years old	–	–	4.8	–	(5.0)	4.3	4.7
21-25 years old	5.8	5.1	4.7	(5.7)	(4.3)	4.4	4.9
26-30 years old	5.7	5.2	4.7	(5.8)	(5.5)	(4.0)	5.1
31-40 years old	5.4	5.2	4.4	5.5	(4.6)	(4.7)	4.8
41-50 years old	4.6	5.1	4.4	(4.0)	4.2	4.2	4.5
51-60 years old	4.9	4.7	3.9	–	4.2	(3.5)	4.1
$>$ 60 years old	(1.7)	(3.3)	(2.5)	–	1.7	(3.3)	2.5
All ages	5.0	5.0	4.3	5.2	4.3	4.1	4.6
No. of respondents	54	121	277	17	67	31	567
No answer	1	3	15	0	6	2	27

(Parentheses indicate that the number of respondents is so small that the value cannot be included in the results, i.e. 5 respondents)

Evaluations by office and maintenance staff have low values—somewhat above 'not especially attractive' (3.2 and 3.1 per cent, respectively). Other nursing staff show the lowest average value—somewhat below 'not especially attractive' (2.8 per cent). The median values for the different groups are in agreement with the average values (see Table 4.7). If the different personnel groups are compared in terms of age, the results are similar to those of the preceding question, though variations are greater.

These answers indicate that ancillary professionals, doctors, and nurses evaluate alternative job possibilities as relatively more attractive than do other groups. As in the preceding question, these three groups evaluate their market position as somewhat more favourable than that of main-

66

Mean value of answers to the question: How attractive would another job be for you?

Age group	Doctors	Nurses	Non-professional nursing staff	Ancillary professional staff	Maintenance and other staff	Office staff	All personnel
< 21 years old	—	—	3.2	—	(3.0)	2.5	3.1
21-25 years old	4.2	4.3	3.0	(4.7)	(3.7)	4.4	3.7
26-30 years old	3.7	4.2	3.2	(3.8)	(4.3)	(4.0)	3.8
31-40 years old	4.5	3.7	2.8	5.2	2.8	(4.3)	3.4
41-50 years old	3.7	4.0	2.9	(3.5)	3.5	3.3	3.2
51-60 years old	3.0	2.7	2.5	—	2.7	(2.3)	2.6
> 60 years old	(2.0)	(2.0)	(1.5)	—	(1.7)	(2.3)	1.9
All ages	3.8	3.8	2.8	4.4	3.1	3.2	3.2
No. of respondents	54	121	277	17	67	31	567
No answer	1	9	13	0	5	1	29

tenance, office and non-professional nursing staff.

A control question was formulated as follows: 'Do you think that measures are required so that the hospital can obtain sufficiently qualified personnel in the future to handle the type of tasks you perform?' Answers to this question, i.e. the employee's own conception of his market position, conform relatively well to the data derived from vacancy statistics.

We said earlier that the interests of different personnel groups are somewhat contradictory. Resolution of conflicts within the hospital is not always handled by the hospital management but sometimes takes place directly between the parties concerned. The most striking example of direct negotiations was between junior doctors and the department chiefs.

67

In this instance, the department chiefs can be regarded as representing the hospital management and are responsible for protecting the interests of other participant groups such as the patients. But department chiefs and junior doctors obviously have conflicting interests on a number of issues. Conditions vary greatly from one department to the next because of the physicians' personal goals, the resources available, and the patients' needs. Table 4.8 was constructed on the basis of statements made by several doctors and does not apply to all departments at General Hospital. But according to the doctors, the table provides a good picture of the conditions in some of the clinical departments.

It is difficult to understand the power of the department chiefs and junior doctors in terms of their demands. To begin with, the 'balance of power' depends to a large extent on the legitimacy of their demands. For example, the department chiefs at General Hospital find it almost im-

TABLE 4.8

Some examples of issues in which department chiefs and junior doctors have conflicting interests.

	Department chiefs want	Junior doctors want
Distribution of workload	Junior physicians to work primarily with in-patients (in patient care is the hospital's main task, this gives department chiefs more time for outpatient care)	Time over for outpatient care (extra income, education)
Working hours	No fixed working hours for junior doctors (makes them more easily available, reduces planning problems)	Fixed working hours
On-call service	Each clinical department to have its own on-call service (reduces pressure on department chiefs' stand by workload, provides better service to patients)	On-call service for several departments combined (reduces on-call workload for junior doctors)[22]

68

possible to enforce their demand that each clinical department provide its own on-call service because they want to lessen the pressure on back-up service, i.e. their own workload. But the department chiefs' medical authority in this instance provides them with substantial opportunities to resist the junior doctors' demands for shared duty.

Other demands made by junior doctors include instruction and guidance, share in outpatient clinics, convenient holiday times, etc. The junior doctors have two important factors in their favour when it comes to realising these demands: market position and their own informal information system.[23] A department chief at General Hospital who does not give his junior doctors a reasonable share of patient fees runs the risk of being boycotted. Several chiefs openly admit that this can occur: 'A department chief's power is very restricted. The junior doctors can boycott me if I don't adhere to the rules of the game. But lately I've had no trouble in finding substitutes.' Many junior doctors say that before they apply for a job they call their colleagues who have worked in the same department and 'get the story'. Several department chiefs make use of former junior doctors who have worked in their departments to help them recruit new junior physicians. Substitutes we met often said that they had 'heard the department was a good one'.

The department chiefs' chances of resisting the demands of junior doctors are based on a number of factors: they distribute tasks, working facilities, and secretarial assistance, and give grades and write references which influence later appointments as department chief.[24]

The situation regarding re-appointment does not only apply to the doctor's own hospital. The department chiefs' association often has a great deal of influence on appointments, although decisions cannot always be based on personal knowledge of the applicant. Colleagues (i.e. other department chiefs) are often contacted to find out about a candidate. Similarly, the department chiefs at General Hospital are often consulted with respect to appointments at other hospitals.

The hospital's relations with its participants—the contribution-inducement balance

The county council

The county council is the hospital's 'owner'. The limits and medical activities of the county council are described in chapter 3 (Fig. 3.8). The contribution-inducement balance at General Hospital was summarised in

69

Table 4.2. The county council provides money to the hospital from tax revenues. The hospital's allotment amounted to 30 million cr. in 1965 (almost a quarter of the county council's total operating budget). Thirty million cr.—or one-third of the county council's total investment expenditure during the last five-year period—1960-65—have gone to General Hospital.

The county council also provides General Hospital with important services such as the School of Nursing associated with the hospital. The staff of the county council organisation department, construction engineers, wages secretary, education and other experts all give advice and carry out studies for the various county agencies. As far as General Hospital is concerned, however, these services (with the exception of the School of Nursing) do not amount to more than one man year per year. But, due to their highly specialised nature, they are still very valuable. This situation is somewhat similar to the relations between an industrial firm's central staff offices and its local administrative personnel.

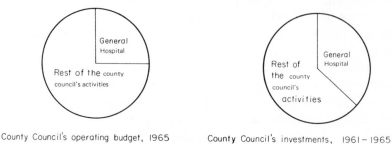

County Council's operating budget, 1965   County Council's investments, 1961–1965

Fig. 4.5   Operating and capital appropriations from the county council.

The most important inducement that the county council receives from General Hospital is 'the voters' goodwill. For obvious reasons, it is difficult to measure this goodwill quantitatively. Since there are hardly any conflicts of opinion between the various political parties over public health and medical care, politicians do not tend to refer to their performance in this area as merits at election time.

There have only been a few instances of sharp criticism of the present county council's performance with regard to health care in Industry Town. The most serious criticism concerned the closure of various units at times. The county council has thus been criticised for poor planning and insufficient efforts in educating the medical staff. Although criticism is not directed at General Hospital itself, but at the council administration, the county council still takes this into account in its evaluation of, and

70

planning for, the hospital. When the leading members of council and its top employees are asked what they think about the management at General Hospital (i.e. the hospital director, chief of the medical staff, and the board of trustees) one of their most unanimous opinions is that greater efforts should be made to recruit and deploy personnel effectively and in general, make good use of the resources at the hospital's disposal, particularly with respect to keeping the nursing units open. But these opinions are not shared by everyone. Some people in the county council readily blame personnel difficulties on conditions outside the control of the hospital. 'Not much can be said about staff problems. It's the same everywhere you turn.'

Our attempts to take an inventory of the county council's unsatisfied demands on General Hospital did not provide much information. Demands for cost reductions or increased efficiency were seldom mentioned and unclearly stated. None of the parties—including the party which had proposed tax cuts—demanded a reduction in appropriations to General Hospital. The county tax was 6 cr. per 100 in 1965 (national average 5.95). In addition to demanding increased efforts to use resources effectively, most people interviewed felt that waiting time in the out-patient clinics was too long. Other than this, the only information we could obtain was that some of the interviewees were with all due respect, critical of the way in which certain clinical departments were run. The demands that General Hospital lessen patients' waiting time at outpatient clinics and that the department chiefs introduce an appointment system have thus far only been expressed as general inquiries from the county council to the department chiefs, via the board of trustees.

The hospital board has a complete and correct picture of the county council's wishes. 'They think we should be able to recruit more nurses.' 'They think we close certain units too often.' 'They are dissatisfied with the waiting lists to get into the hospital, and the waiting time at the outpatient clinics.' 'They aren't satisfied with the way some of the departments are run.' 'They think we should manage our personnel situation more effectively.' These statements are quoted from our records of interviews with the hospital's management. Identical statements were made by leading members and representatives of the county council.

Since we were interested in these demands on General Hospital, which were expressed by the county council, we tried to find out how the county council gives priority to different demands. We found that leading council members and representatives (Social Democrats, as well as the other parties) think that the voters' demands for the best possible care predominate. Demands for cost reductions and efficiency should not be

71

ranked ahead of the demand for quality. The long waiting lists and lack of personnel often tend to give the highest priority to the demand that the hospital keep functioning. There is a committee whose job is to investigate ways of saving money. The records of this committee include one of the most consciously formulated deliberations as to how different demands should be ranked. At this committee's first meeting it was decided that 'the first goal should be to solve the capacity problem in the health sector'.

The hospital's unsatisfied demands are also rather limited. Dissatisfaction mostly arises because the hospital's facilities have not been expanded. Some results of this delay are that facilities at the department of infectious diseases are unsatisfactory, and certain new specialties such as pathology and bacteriology have not been established despite the urgent requests of the department chiefs and the board at General Hospital over the years. In connection with their latest refusal to appropriate funds, the county council said that a new long-term plan was required first. Many people at General Hospital interpreted this as an unnecessary pretext for delay.

We made a detailed study of the budgeting process during a three-year period to ascertain the amount and type of requests denied. The budget for 1965 can be used as a typical example. The hospital requested 28.2 million cr. This meant that certain demands from department chiefs were not included (see Table 4.4). The health and medical services board approved a budget of 27.9 million cr., which was granted by the county council. The difference included 250,000 cr. for salaries and 90,000 cr. for other costs. The reduction was not made on the basis of factual information, but was due to a pessimistic evaluation about filling certain vacancies and a more cautious estimate of various costs.

The hospital also requested an appropriation to the capital budget amounting to 1.25 million cr. This sum was lower than the amount requested by the department chiefs.[25] The county council granted 0.96 million cr. The 0.29 million cr. that it refused to grant was intended for a new X-ray laboratory, and for an automatic rotating-card index for the surgery department. The first project (amounting to 0.27 million cr.) was rejected on the grounds that appropriations had recently been made for re-equipping the existing X-ray laboratory. The other request was rejected because the council thought that an investigation was required to determine the most suitable equipment.

In this request for appropriations in the following year the X-ray department chief did not mention the previous request. The chief of the medical staff told us that 'as far as equipment which can be bought is

72

concerned the county council is very obliging. When it comes to establishing new positions we are supposed to aim at conformity, which implies a certain amount of restriction.'

Most people in responsible positions at General Hospital and the county council administration had unanimous and clear opinions about what the hospital needed. But most of the council members interviewed had unclear, incomplete, and sometimes even erroneous conceptions of 'the most important requirements requested by General Hospital but not yet granted by the county council'. For instance, one member said: 'There have been no new requests from the clinical departments but they do want to expand facilities.' Another mentioned 'the employees' dining-room', and a third, 'planning for certain jobs, such as secretaries' as being foremost on the list of unsatisfied demands.

Even when the department chiefs were asked 'what are the most important resource requirements requested by General Hospital but not yet granted by the county council?', their answers did not amount to a forbidding list of demands. Five out of fifteen chiefs said that their appropriations do not cover the facilities they require. The shortages mentioned included office aids such as intercoms, box-conveyor systems, dictaphones; also automation equipment, a swimming pool for a specific department, etc.

Thus, it is hardly surprising that neither General Hospital nor the county council has deliberated on more radical measures aimed at regulating the other party. Six long-serving members of the county council answered the following question negatively: 'Has there to your knowledge been any discussion in the county council, its offices, or agencies during the past few years with regard to a significant reorganisation of General Hospital for the purpose of increasing efficiency or changing the objectives of its activities?' Some of the respondents mentioned that establishment of the jobs of hospital director, chief nurse and nursing supervisor involved substantial organisational changes. But they quickly added that no other organisational intervention had been discussed. The following quotation is from our records of an interview during which the above question was asked:

Well, yes ... not exactly .... When we appointed the hospital director we did discuss these matters .... If other powers could be assigned to him afterwards .... Heavy demands are made on him .... He has to be firm and flexible at the same time ....We have to have a hospital director who is apart from the physicians—otherwise their position becomes too strong. This means hiring top people in the

73

field. Remember that as far as size is concerned we're talking about an organisation as large as the Grängesberg company.[26]

When the hospital's management and department chiefs were asked a similar question their answers were just as negative. 'Sometimes state or local agencies make use of press campaigns, etc. to try to influence the authorities responsible for granting appropriations.' When asked whether 'power measures' such as these had been discussed by the department chiefs' association, or groups of department chiefs, all respondents agreed that this had not occurred.

We observed some elements of formal conflict between the hospital's management and the county council. Some public statements contained complaints that the prescribed means of providing information and making decisions were not always applied. This matter now seems to have been cleared up, and the various parties have adjusted their actions accordingly. Perhaps the only thing remaining is a desire on the part of the hospital's management to 'be better informed'.

Patients

The patients are the hospital's clients or customers, i.e. 'production' at the hospital is aimed at satisfying the needs of this participant group. Figure 4.2 (the contribution-inducement balance) showed that the patient makes few direct contributions to the hospital but places great demands on it. Conditions differ somewhat, depending on whether the patient receives in-patient or outpatient care. But since these two overlap to some extent, they will be dealt with as one unit.

Patients (almost 16,000 in-patients and slightly more than 47,000 out-patients in 1965) pay a fee of 5 cr. (1965) as their daily charge and most important direct contribution. The national social insurance usually covers this fee for in-patients (by deducting it from benefits to be paid to the patient). Outpatients pay between 7 and 30 cr. per visit, of which 1.60, and in some instances slightly more, goes to the hospital, the rest to the physician. In special cases, outpatients have to pay even higher fees. Patients admitted to semi-private or private rooms also pay a fee (15 and 30 cr., respectively) intended to cover extra 'hotel costs'.[27]

From the patient's point of view it is much more advantageous to be admitted to the hospital. In some areas, such as the rehabilitation department, the doctor can choose between outpatient or in-patient care. The former implies much lower costs for the hospital while the fees paid by

74

the patients are significantly higher.[28]

One example concerned a patient involved in a traffic accident. First he was admitted to the department of surgery. Later, he was moved to the rehabilitation department. The doctor in charge had to decide whether the patient should remain hospitalised or be treated at home by a visiting nurse. The patient requested hospitalisation because he had difficulty in arranging care at home. Assuming a three-week period of treatment including, at least in the beginning, daily medical surveillance, the cost to the taxpayer of hospitalising this patient could be estimated at 600 cr., and care at home, between 100 and 300 cr. Thus, in the first case, the cost to the patient would be nothing, and in the latter, 300-600 cr. Differences between the hospital's and patients' costs are often even greater.

The inducements requested and received by most patients are diagnosis, treatment, and care. These services are often very expensive. For instance, the average cost to the hospital in 1965 was 40 cr. per outpatient and 104 cr. per in-patient. Later, when the complexities of the products are studied in more detail, the large discrepancies between different departments become more apparent.

Differences between individual patients are even greater but cost accounting at the hospital was incomplete so that we could not obtain precise information about the costs for each. The high costs associated with a complicated case are shown in Table 5.3. Some patients are given special benefits. But less than 1 per cent were admitted to semi-private or private rooms. Some 6.3 per cent of in-patients and 10.7 per cent of outpatients were treated as emergencies, i.e. given immediate care without waiting.

A fairly large number of patients make special demands on the hospital, the biggest group being those who need health certificates. (This is described in detail in chapter 5 in connection with the hospital's products.) Patients whose only errand to the hospital involves certificates amount to nearly 5 per cent of the total number of patients in some departments, though much less in others. In the chest clinic and paediatric department for example, medical check-ups are an important part of the activities, as compared with most other departments, in which they are rare.

When the institutions for resolving conflicts between the hospital and patients were described, we said that the hospital has an almost absolute, and wholly legitimate, monopoly position. There are only two ways in which the patients can assert their unsatisfied demands on the hospital— collectively, via negotiations and pressure on decision-making authorities, and via the complaint procedure. We tried to make a list of the demands presented collectively by voters or patient groups to the following bodies:

75

1 Political party groups in the county council.
2 The county council.
3 The county council executive committee and the health and medical services board.
4 Staff offices of the county council.
5 The hospital's board of trustees.
6 The hospital director and the chief of the medical staff.

The results were surprisingly scant. The demands made to the county council almost exclusively related to expanding health care, and not to General Hospital or its functions. The only type of demand presented to these authorities which had to do with General Hospital was related to waiting time at the outpatient clinics. Individuals, groups, and patient groups in various patient organisations, have all tried to influence changes in this area. In one instance, a group of patients with regularly recurring needs for tests tried to enlist the cooperation of the county council for an arrangement involving priority in the outpatient clinic.

Our investigation with regard to the complaint procedure produced equally few results. We expected to find some kind of 'complaint funnel', i.e. a reduction in number as complaints reach successively higher levels of authority, since most complaints are rejected, or lead to measures at a lower level. Our interviews did confirm our expectations at the clinical level. But the situation is different above the level of department chief. Above this, the authorities have no real power until we reach the National Board of Health and Welfare and the courts. When deliberating whether or not to complain, patients are already (or become) aware of this situation. They find out that if their complaints are to lead to some kind of action, the whole complaint procedure has to be gone through until they reach the superior authorities.

The very limited number of complaints is just as interesting as the complaint procedure itself.[29] The small amount of complaints is probably explained by the following two factors: (a) either all the hospital's patients are completely satisfied with the care and service they receive; or (b) they cannot, do not want to, dare not, or think that it is not worthwhile to complain. Knowledge as to which of these two explanations is correct is extremely interesting from other points of view. It is probably less important so far as the hospital and its management are concerned. As we said before, the only time a patient actually has a chance to assert his demands is when his complaint can be reported to the National Board of Health and Welfare.

76

The hospital management

The hospital management comprises those people responsible for running the hospital in conformity with objectives formulated by the owners (the county council). Everyone on the county council and its staff thinks that this definition implies that the hospital management constitutes the following: the board of trustees, the hospital director, and the chief of the medical staff. The board of trustees has seven representatives and several deputy members, one of whom also participates regularly. The board is chosen by the county council, and reflects party representation in the council. Thus, the chairman is a Social Democrat, and the vice-chairman a Liberal. The chief of medical staff is head of one of the hospital's clinical departments, and the hospital director is an economist. At least ten department chiefs attend board meetings regularly. Additional information about the hospital management is given in Figs. 4.6 and 4.7 and Table 4.9.

Among those who comprise the hospital management, the hospital director has a unique position with respect to contributions and inducements. This is primarily because he is the only full-time management employee. His working week is more than 50 hours long. The chief of the medical staff and chairman of the board devote somewhat less time to management activities. Their total workload varies a great deal during the year, from a half-time job to two or three hours per week. These three,

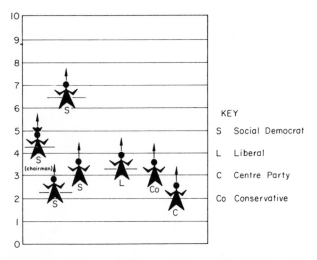

KEY

S Social Democrat

L Liberal

C Centre Party

Co Conservative

Fig. 4.6 Political status of the members of the board of trustees at General Hospital.[30]

77

along with the vice-chairman, have a heavier workload than the other board members because they are also members of the executive subcommittee. The board and subcommittee each meet about once a month. These meetings are usually held in the afternoon or evening and last an average of four to five hours (subcommittee) and one or two hours (board).

The only economic inducement for these contributions to the hospital is a fixed salary or a fee. The hospital director apart, board members receive little remuneration (see Table 4.10). Nor are there any significant indirect economic inducements involved, the possible exception being that members of the board think that they receive more personal medical attention if they happen to require it. 'I've been sick myself a couple of times and it's obvious that I can come and go much more freely than an average patient.' 'Contacts with department chiefs have been valuable and stimulating.' According to the members and others, participation on the

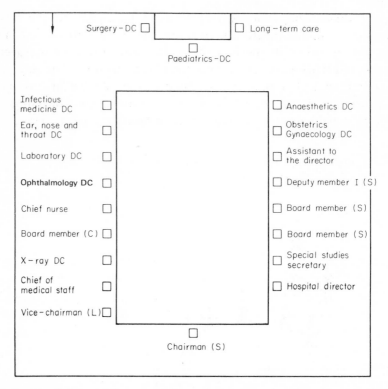

Fig. 4.7 Participants in a meeting of the board of trustees at General Hospital (DC = department chief; S = Social Democrat; L = Liberal; C = Centre Party).

78

TABLE 4.9

Experience of the board of trustees at General Hospital

Party distribution	4 Social Democrats 1 Centre Party 1 Liberal 1 Conservative
No. of years on the board	Maximum, 13 years Average, 7 years Minimum, 1 year
Other leadership experience in large organisations or firms	Half the members have such experience

hospital board is not a stepping-stone to appointment in other positions. This was also confirmed by a look at the current jobs of those who had previously belonged to the board.

Thus, rather small economic inducements are linked with membership of the hospital board. The chief of the medical staff's fee is only a fraction of a junior doctor's income for the same number of hours of work in a clinic. But several members feel that the fee is not worse, and sometimes better, than amounts paid for other positions of trust. We received similar answers to the following question: 'Do you think that measures are required to recruit qualified people to perform your task on the board in the future?' Respondents said that 'reasonable compensation' is necessary, i.e. an 'increase in the *per diem* fee'. It is also interesting to note that more than half the members think that some specific education should be required for those serving on the board.

Membership of the hospital's board is regarded as an interesting and stimulating task. Five of the seven members believe that it is better, or much better, than other positions of trust. But none gave any clear indication of their most significant duties in this respect. Half said that they had another more important community, union, or business activity. The most satisfying thing about working on the board seems to be contact with an important public function. Cooperation within the board is also regarded as a positive ingredient (more than half the members have been on the board for more than six years). The elements giving most dissatisfaction were difficulties in conjunction with the hospital's personnel problems, and a lack of influence on the management of the hospital as a whole.

Assessment of the board's unsatisfied demands on the hospital yielded

79

TABLE 4.10

Approximate working time and economic inducement for the hospital board members

	Approximate working time devoted to hospital management (excluding travel time)	Economic compensation (Swedish crowns)	Compensation per hour of work (excluding travel time)
Hospital director	55 hours/week	Salary grade[31] KB1 — 53,928/year	30/hour
Chief of the medical staff	2-20 hours/week	10,000/year	20/hour
Chairman of the board	2—10 hours/week	5,000/year +50/meeting	30/hour
Vice-chairman	2—6 hours/meeting	50 tot 65/ meeting	15/hour
Members 1—6	2—4 hours/ meeting 8—10 times/ year	50 tot 65/ meeting	15 to 30 depending on time spent in preparation

the same results as the hospital's unsatisfied demands on the board. The board believes that its position is too weak and that economic benefits are not commensurate with the amount of responsibility or working time involved. On the other hand, dissatisfaction has not been strong enough to motivate countermeasures, and only one person contemplated leaving the board within the next three years.

We assessed the views of the county council and the board as to the latter's management contributions to the hospital. The responses can be divided into two groups. The main question asked was: 'Do you think the management at General Hospital (we refer to the hospital director, chief of the medical staff, and the board of trustees) should make any additional contributions?' A number of related questions were also included.

One group of respondents (several of whom were currently serving on

80

the board) based their answers on their own views of what is required for the hospital to function well. Their evaluation was that the hospital board lacked resources, and functioned unsatisfactorily. The board was regarded as too large, especially as all department chiefs participate in the meetings. The subcommittee was unanimously felt to be a unit which functions much better: 'The political representatives don't have enough time to devote themselves to the hospital's problems, and meetings usually only deal with insignificant, routine matters which the county council ultimately decides anyway.'

'Hospital and county council legislation should probably be different. Work on the board is more unwieldy than in a local government committee or board. We should be able to assume more responsibility. Our responsibility right now is plus or minus zero. The hospital board's position in relation to the county council is too weak for us to assert ourselves with respect to hospital personnel. Our resources are not sufficient for managing a hospital of this size.' The chief of the medical staff in particular is critical of his sphere of influence: 'If I were a director I would have greater authority. But I would rather devote myself to developing my department and other similar clinical departments in the country. The job of chief of the medical staff conflicts too much with my work as a doctor. It's an impossible job. And it consumes all my leisure time.' Other interviewees also felt that a physician was needed to deal with hospital management problems on a full-time basis.

The second group of respondents based their answers on the hospital board's present resources and position—according to law and custom. Their evaluations refer only to how well the management functions given the possibilities allowed by prevailing conditions. The result was that this group expressed unanimous confidence in all members of the hospital board. We tried to measure relations more precisely by giving interviewees a list of the ten board members, and asking the following:

Here is a list of the ten members of the hospital board . . . . Assume hospital legislation prescribed that appointments to the board be approved by the county council. If you were a member of council how many of these persons would you recommend for appointment?

All respondents expressed their confidence in all ten persons.

The department chiefs

As hospital participants, the department chiefs belong to the 'employee' group. Their importance with regard to management of the hospital will be described in chapter 6. At present, we are interested in their contributions as employees of the hospital, the inducements that they request in return, and the extent to which they can assert their demands.

The most important contribution of the hospital's sixteen department chiefs is an exceedingly long working week. Information based on diaries kept during a fourteen-day period indicated that 48 hours is the average time worked, with an average of three hours' evening work per week. As a rule, department chiefs are not required to be on call to the same extent as junior doctors. On the other hand, most department chiefs—sometimes in rota with their assistants—constantly have to serve on a stand-by basis at home. This implies being available for telephone consultations and being called to the hospital on short notice, though most department chiefs are not called out very often. Figure 4.8 shows the large differences in the workloads of different doctors.

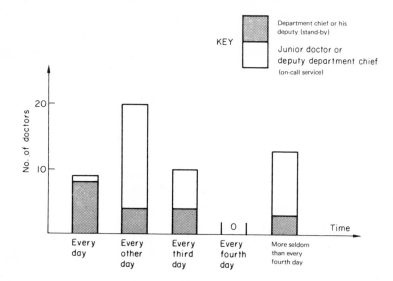

Fig. 4.8   On-call workload of doctors at General Hospital.

There are several reasons for these differences. The doctors themselves say that some departments are 'busier'. A large number of junior doctors—and success in filling these positions with experienced junior doctors—are prerequisites for limiting one's own workload. A small

82

number of nursing units also means less work. The number and type of patients treated in the outpatient clinics are most important, and to some extent, easiest to regulate. This is probably the most significant source of variations in the workload.

The department chiefs' most important inducement for their contributions to the hospital is a fixed salary, and for most, an opportunity to earn extra income from the outpatient clinics.[32] The relation between working time in outpatient clinics and annual income is shown in Fig. 4.9. Most of the doctors themselves regulate their income from outpatient care. The influx to the hospital is so great that every available hour a doctor has is taken up by patients.

The department chiefs believe that conditions at General Hospital are more or less comparable with those in other hospitals. Another relevant comparison is with executives whose salaries are closely related to their 'ranking in the hierarchy'. The department chiefs' position was thought comparable to that of executives in large or medium-sized firms in Industry Town; in other words, the department chiefs are among the town's 'bigwigs'.

Most department chiefs (15 out of 16) regard their jobs as permanent and are generally satisfied with the inducements they receive from the hospital. 'Of course, most of our salary goes to taxes—and remember, we can't make very many deductions. We can't even travel to a convention without having to pay for it ourselves.' The department chiefs' union—the Association of Hospital Doctors—also makes rather modest demands on the hospital. Sometimes, certain doctors who are treated unfavourably request improvements. The doctors do not complain about working time; instead they prefer to make advantageous comparisons to the way things were in the past. Many decide to work long hours of their own free will. Several assured us: 'I work primarily because I like to.'

New demands from the department chiefs are usually aimed at the county council and not the hospital. They do not request personal benefits but, rather, improved resources for their departments, e.g. an extra junior doctor, social worker, nursing units, grants for new equipment, improved facilities, an assistant department chief in a subspecialty, better bacteriological and pathological services, etc. Of course, it is more realistic to include personal motives as part of these demands for better resources. In any case, the department chiefs and the hospital's management are frank enough to admit that demands (such as annual requests for grants) are sometimes based on personal motives. They also feel that administrative matters could be handled more smoothly and rapidly.

The absence of unsatisfied demands is also reflected in our direct

83

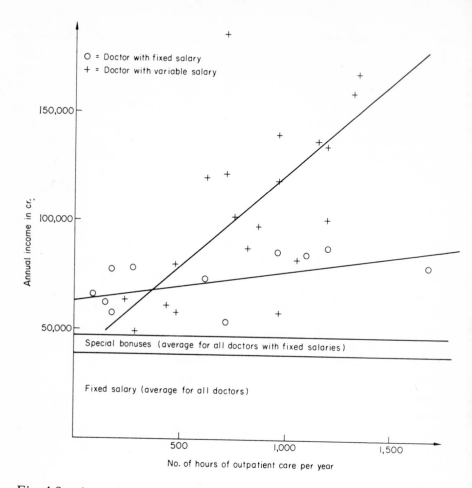

O = Doctor with fixed salary
+ = Doctor with variable salary

Annual income in cr.

150,000

100,000

50,000

Special bonuses (average for all doctors with fixed salaries)

Fixed salary (average for all doctors)

500   1,000   1,500

No. of hours of outpatient care per year

Fig. 4.9   Annual income and working time of doctors in the outpatient units at General Hospital.[33]

measurements of various relations based on different kinds of statistics. Turnover among department chiefs is very low; during the past ten-year period only one department chief has left the hospital for reasons other than retirement. Next year (1966), the primary reason for leaving can be expected to be retirement (12 out of 16), even though most (10 out of 16) think that it would be easy, or even very easy, to obtain another, equivalent job, and that these are fairly attractive or even very attractive (5 out of 16) (see Tables 4.6 and 4.25).

It is difficult to obtain specific information on demands in the opposite direction, i.e. demands made by the hospital on the department chiefs as employees. There were no particularly strong reactions on the part of the

84

hospital board, or members and representatives of the county council to the following questions: 'Would you want one or more of the department chiefs to make contributions to General Hospital that he/they do not make at present?' and 'Would you want one or more of the department chiefs to work differently in some respect from the way he/they work today?' The minor criticism arising as a result of these questions did not by any means refer to the department chiefs as a whole.

On the basis of our experience of industrial firms, we expected the hospital management to complain because the department chiefs did not identify sufficiently with the hospital and the county council in situations in which they were obvious representatives of the hospital. In fact, we found that the department chiefs often identified with junior staff and even patients, against the hospital. On the other hand, no one in the hospital management ever expressed this point of view spontaneously. When we mentioned what we had observed, people agreed with us, though they were not disturbed or surprised.[34]

To obtain more specific measurements of the relations between the hospital and the department chiefs, we put the following question to the twelve people on the board and the county council who were said to know the doctors best:

> Here is a list of the 16 department chiefs at General Hospital. Assume that department chiefs are only appointed for a period of three years with the possibility of reappointment. How many of these chiefs would you recommend for reappointment?

The response indicated that an average of 12.5 would have been re-appointed.

Other personnel

An employee's most important contribution to the hospital is his work. This is usually measured in terms of working time,[35] even though this measurement is often imperfect (see Fig. 4.10). Junior doctors and top administrative personnel work longer than other staff. The average working week for junior doctors and top administrative personnel is about 55 and 50 hours, respectively. The normal working week for other staff is about 45 hours. Nurses often work overtime, particularly at certain times of the year.

Table 4.11 shows that some personnel groups make 'additional contri-

85

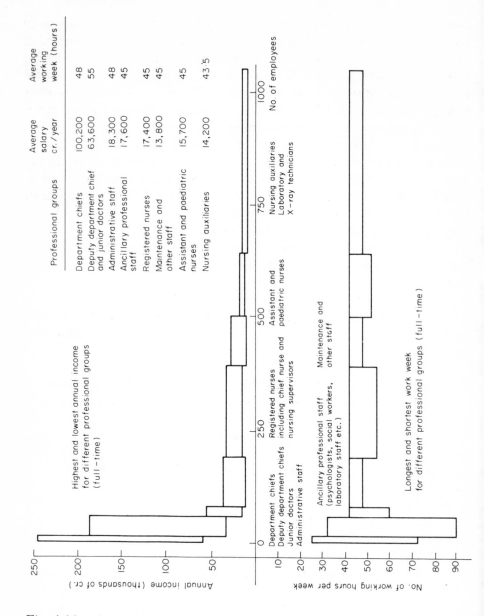

Professional groups	Average salary cr./year	Average working week (hours)
Department chiefs	100,200	48
Deputy department chief and junior doctors	63,600	55
Administrative staff	18,300	48
Ancillary professional staff	17,600	45
Registered nurses	17,400	45
Maintenance and other staff	13,800	45
Assistant and paediatric nurses	15,700	45
Nursing auxiliaries	14,200	43.5

Fig. 4.10 Annual income and working hours per week for full-time employees.

butions' primarily in terms of on-call service, shifts, and other forms of inconvenient working hours. Junior doctors and other groups have the heaviest burden owing to extensive on-call obligations, as do the night

86

staff who begin at 9.30 p.m. and finish at 7.00 a.m. The on-call workload for doctors is shown in Fig. 4.8. Nurses and other medical staff also think that the recurring changes from one working schedule to another, and the division of these schedules into morning and afternoon shifts is a complication (especially for married women). However, our comments in this instance are based wholly on interviews with the hospital management, personnel experts, and representatives of the different personnel organisations.

The employees' main inducement is their pay. Doctors, nurses, administrative personnel, ancillary professional personnel, assistant nurses and nursing auxiliaries receive a fixed salary. Hourly wages are paid to other personnel and temporaries. In addition, most doctors who work in the outpatient clinics receive a *per capita* remuneration from the patients they treat. All personnel, except doctors and some personnel in positions of authority (such as supervisory nurses), receive compensation for overtime. On-call personnel also receive special compensation. Most of the staff who belong to a union exercise their right to cash compensation for overtime (usually 1.5 times their normal hourly wage). Most of the nurses prefer time off in compensation for overtime, as do doctors who are obliged to be on call. The doctors and nurses are generally satisfied with extra time off as compensation for overtime or on-call duty.

Salaries at the hospital are illustrated in Fig. 4.10, and are probably the same as in most industrial firms but higher than in most civil service jobs. In terms of rate per hour, however, salaries are less attractive in that those who receive the highest (i.e. the doctors) usually work longer than other groups. Figure 4.9 shows that two 'income blocs' can be distinguished among the doctors, i.e. physicians with variable salaries (and high income from patients), and physicians with fixed salaries (and no, or insignificant income from patients). Salaries in the former group depend on the number of hours spent in the outpatient clinics. A third group is composed of radiologists and pathologists who have relatively high incomes (average income approximately 175,000 cr. per year in 1965).

Figure 4.11 shows that there is a considerable difference between different doctors' earnings per hour (14–71 cr.). There is another interesting difference between these two income groups. Doctors with 'variable salaries' (i.e. high income from patients) are recorded as devoting many hours to the outpatient clinics, and giving short treatment periods per patient. What kind of relationship exists in this instance? Do short treatment periods (and thus, high earnings per hour) stimulate doctors to spend many hours in the outpatient clinics? Or is the pressure from patient waiting lists so great that it forces the doctors to combine many hours of

87

TABLE 4.11

'Extra contributions' in excess of the normal work day

Personnel group	Special services			
	On-call obligations	Paid overtime (see working schedule Figure 4.10)	Shift duty	Inconvenient working hours
Department chiefs	Stand-by (see Figure 4.8).			
Junior doctors	Most are on-call every other or every third night.			
Nurses and midwives	Some surgical and reception nurses and some midwives.	Ward nurses. Personnel up to salary level KA 19	Day staff alternate every third or fourth week between different schedules. Night duty.	Often for nursing service personnel.
Laboratory staff	Blood-bank personnel on call every third night. The remainder every sixth night.	Personnel up to salary level KA 19		Often for nursing service personnel.
Administrative staff	Some on-call responsibility for chief nurse and nursing	Personnel up to salary level KA 19		Some office staff. work on Saturdays.

88

Table 4.11 (continued)

| Maintenance staff | Some maintenance and repairman. | Personnel up to salary level KA 19 | | Some maintenance staff work on Saturdays. |
| Medical service personnel | Some surgical and reception staff. | Personnel up to salary level KA 19 | Day staff alternate every third or fourth week between different schedules. Night duty. | Often for nursing service personnel. |

work with short treatment times? Most doctors we talked to referred to the latter explanation. But the relationship seems to be the opposite for doctors on 'fixed salaries'. They have long treatment periods per patient, and spend many hours in outpatient clinics.

Table 4.12 shows that the employees receive various extra benefits in addition to their salaries. These benefits differ from one group to the next. Some doctors value opportunities to do research very highly. Priority options on housing, or the possibility of renting flats owned by the hospital are probably also valued highly by all personnel groups.[36] On-the-job educational opportunities are becoming more and more important. We took particular note of the force behind these demands from unregistered nursing personnel and their union.

Appointments and promotions among the various professional groups are summarised in Fig. 4.12. Individual groups seem to be closed, and there have been few promotions from one to another. Appointments and/or promotions usually require extensive further education (or re-education) and training. The most important exception is the promotion of nursing auxiliaries to assistant nurses. The opinions of various persons in the administration and personnel department as to promotion prospects are summarised in Table 4.13. These expectations of future opportunities are consistent with the pattern of promotions which have taken place thus far (see Fig. 4.12). This also conforms to the employees' own views when they were asked about their career plans.

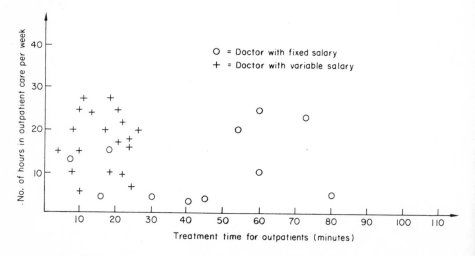

Fig. 4.11 Working time of doctors and the average treatment time per outpatient.

90

TABLE 4.12

'Extra inducement' to personnel at General Hospital in addition to their salaries

Personnel group	Opportunities to do research	On-the-job training	Housing supplied or owned by the hospital	Priority options on housing	Personnel dining-room	Child day-care centres	Foreign travel, conferences, etc.	On-call and overtime compensation
Special benefits								
Department chiefs	(See Table 5.1).	Short special courses.	All personnel have the right to apply for housing in the hospital's personnel residences.	All personnel categories that are difficult to recruit locally have priority options on housing (physiotherapists, social workers, doctors, nurses).	All personnel can buy meal tickets (Breakfast, 1.23 cr.; lunch and supper 2.92 cr.)	There is a day-care centre. Nurses have priority. Demand is greater than supply.	Sometimes.	Extra time off as on-call compensation. Time off or pay for overtime.
Junior doctors		Short special courses.						
Nurses and midwives		Continuing education. Charge nurse course.						
Laboratory staff			Nursing service personnel comprise the largest group living in hospital housing					
Office staff and medical secretaries		Medical secretary course.						
Other professional staff (social workers, physiotherapists)								
Maintenance and other staff								
Nursing service (personnel)		Nursing instructor will be hired. This personnel group, more than any other, uses paid leave of absence for educational puposes.						

91

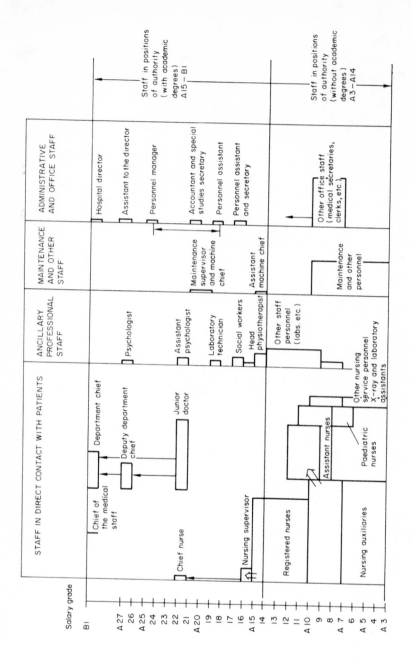

Fig. 4.12　Appointments and promotions within General Hospital.

92

TABLE 4.13

Opinions of some employees at General Hospital as to appointment and/or promotion possibilities

Whoever is	Can in practice be appointed without re-education to the position of	Hospital director	Department chief	Deputy department chief	Assistant to the director	Junior doctor	Hospital accountant	Personnel manager	Personnel assistant	Special studies secretary	Chief nurse	Nursing supervisor	Charge nurse	Registered nurse	Assistant nurse	Paediatric nurse	Janitor	Orderly	Messenger girl/boy
Hospital director																			
Department chief																			
Deputy department chief			x																
Assistant to the director		x																	
Junior doctor			x	x															
Hospital accountant		(x)		x															
Personnel manager																			
Personnel assistant								x											
Special studies secretary		(x)		x															
Chief nurse																			
Nursing supervisor											(x)(x)	x							
Charge nurse											(x)(x)(x)	x							
Registered nurse											(x)(x)(x)(x)	x							
Assistant nurse																			
Paediatric nurse															x				
Janitor																			
Orderly																			
Messenger girl/boy																	x	(x)(x)	

x = occurs fairly often
(x) = rarely occurs

Appointment and/or promotion is not the only purpose of further education. The following informal report from the hospital's management summarises educational efforts during 1965.

Two girls attended a 145-day course for medical secretaries, with pay amounting to salary level KA5. Thirty nurses and other potential supervisors attended a one-week course for supervisors, salary KA14.

93

Two nurses received nursing instructor education for one and a half years, salary KA12 (full salary). Thirteen nursing auxiliaries took a 32-week course for assistant nurses, salary KA7 (full salary). Twenty-six girls attended a course for nursing auxiliaries (of which fifteen went for 23 weeks and eight for 7 weeks-average salary KA5). Four department chiefs were away at courses lasting from three days to a week. Two junior doctors were each gone for one week, and two assistant department chiefs were each away for three days. All these employees received a leave of absence with full salary and compensation for costs of the courses.

Administrative personnel also took part in courses. One personnel assistant attended a two-month course, with salary compensation KA17. Two personnel assistants were each gone for one week to attend a course in personnel organisation. The hospital comptroller participated in a one-week ADP course. Ancillary professional personnel took part in further education as follows: chief social worker, four days; cytology assistant, three days; head physiotherapist, four days; head therapist, two six-day periods. All received full salary and travel expenses.

Many employees at the hospital think that their work in itself is not only a sacrifice but a reward. Our informal conversations with each personnel group all contained assurances that the employees work primarily because they like their work.

We tried to obtain more quantitative information about these conditions by asking: 'What do you think is most satisfying about your working conditions?' The replies are indicated in the right-hand side of Fig. 4.13. The most striking result is the similarity between groups. However, some of the differences are also noteworthy. Doctors indicate that responsibility, independence, and cooperation in their work, i.e. their working role in relation to superiors and colleagues, are the most important factors. Nurses believe that their working role in relation to patients is a primary source of satisfaction. Attitudes of other nursing staff are somewhere between those of nurses and doctors. Ancillary professional staff indicated even more clearly than did the doctors that responsibility, independence, and cooperation were most important. Maintenance staff were the only group that fairly frequently mentioned their convenient working hours as an important factor.

These differences in primary sources of satisfaction between various employee categories are hardly suprising in terms of the way their working roles are designed. The answers are also consistent with the responses to a

94

question about the weight assigned to different types of contacts in order to attain job satisfaction. Table 4.14 shows that doctors give the lowest ranking to contact with patients; contacts with colleagues are much more important. Non-professional nursing staff probably rank contacts with patients higher than the nurses do because they consistently give doctors the lowest ranking.

TABLE 4.14

Most important types of contacts for attaining job satisfaction

What types of contacts are the most important for you *to feel satisfied in your work*? Indicate what you think is most important by 1, next in importance by 2, etc.

	Mean values of ranking given by		
	Doctors	Nurses	Non-professional nursing staff
getting along well with the patients	1.94	1.78	1.74
getting along well with the doctors	1.64	2.05	2.77
getting along well with the nurses	2.12	2.04	1.76
getting along well with the nursing auxiliaries	3.23	1.83	1.93

Unsatisfied demands of the personnel

Our own preliminary interviews, and some carried out by the management consultants commissioned by the hospital's administration indicated that the employees' most important unsatisfied demands, with respect to their employer, involved dissatisfaction with salaries, Industry Town, their supervisors, or the working team to which they belonged. The personnel were asked in a questionnaire: 'What do you find most dissatisfying about your work and working conditions?' The answers are indicated on the left-hand side of Fig. 4.13. For doctors the main source of dissatisfaction was their long working hours and fast work pace ('always in a hurry'). This factor was also important for the registered nurses, who were equally dissatisfied by poor contact, lack of independence, and staff shortages. The most serious sources of dissatisfaction for other non-professional nursing staff were external working conditions and physically heavy work.

Some persons in each of the personnel categories also mentioned what they thought were defects in the hospital's organisation and policies (such as poor working schedules, incomplete information, etc.). But these factors were not a predominant source of dissatisfaction. This also applied to salaries, which were mentioned by only a few interviewees.

Dissatisfaction with salary

In addition to the open question about sources of dissatisfaction we asked the employees to evaluate their working conditions in various ways. Since dissatisfaction with salary is usually linked to comparisons of one's own salary with that of other comparable individuals or groups, we asked employees at General Hospital to indicate whether they thought that others at the hospital, or on the labour market in general, received higher salaries even though their jobs were less demanding or carried less responsibility. It should be noted that, by mistake, only department chiefs and not all doctors were questioned. Table 4.15 shows that there are no large employee groups who feel they are treated unfairly in relation to others at General Hospital.[37] But about half the nurses and ancillary professional staff think that certain employees receive better pay even though their jobs carry less responsibility. Registered nurses mentioned groups such as physiotherapists, assistant nurses, and nursing auxiliaries in reference to age allowances and the salaries of office staff. Physiotherapists are mentioned the most by the social workers.

The hospital staff are generally less satisfied with their situation in comparisons between themselves and the labour market in general (see Table 4.16). Again, registered nurses and ancillary professional staff are the least satisfied. About half the people in these groups feel that many other professional workers receive unwarranted advantages which they themselves do not receive. They also make comparisons with such varied groups as teachers, office staff, and factory and construction workers. It is interesting to note that non-professional nursing and maintenance staff express less dissatisfaction in their answers than do nurses. Most people in these two groups do not think that they are treated unfairly compared

96

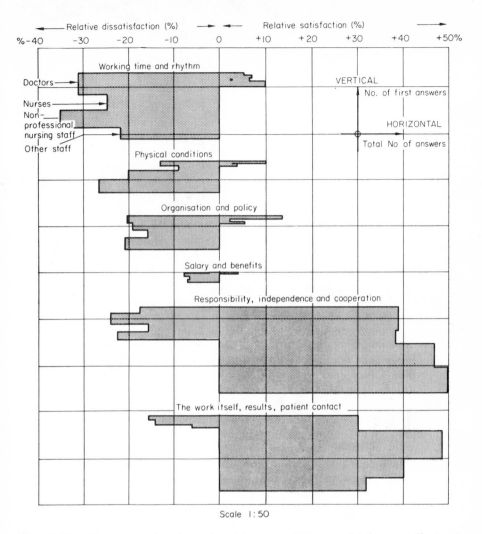

Relative dissatisfaction (%) ⟶   ⟵ Relative satisfaction (%) ⟶

%-40   -30   -20   -10   0   +10   +20   +30   +40   +50%

Working time and rhythm

Doctors

Nurses

Non-professional nursing staff

Other staff

VERTICAL
No. of first answers

HORIZONTAL
Total No of answers

Physical conditions

Organisation and policy

Salary and benefits

Responsibility, independence and cooperation

The work itself, results, patient contact

Scale 1:50

Fig. 4.13   Factors related to working conditions which contribute to satisfaction and dissatisfaction.

with other groups in society. Some department chiefs say that other doctors are better paid even though they perform less demanding tasks with less responsibility. Maintenance staff mention office personnel and porters as favoured groups. Department chiefs mention industrial executives and businessmen in comparisons with the labour market in general. Maintenance staff feel that they are treated unfavourably in comparisons with factory workers, sales and office staff.

97

TABLE 4.15

'Salary envy' within General Hospital

Are there groups of employees at General Hospital whose salaries are higher than yours even though their jobs are less demanding and carry less responsibility?

	Department chiefs (%)	Nurses (%)	Non-professional nursing staff (%)	Ancillary professional staff (%)	Maintenance and other staff (%)	Office staff (%)
Yes, many (3)	0	7	7	6	10	7
Yes, certain groups (2)	19	42	10	65	11	26
No, not as far as I know (1)	81	50	83	29	79	66
No. of respondents	16	121	277	17	67	31
No answer	0	12	21	0	3	4
If yes, which groups do you mean?	Other doctors	Other professional groups	Other similar professional groups	Other professional groups often in the same part of the hospital	Very different answers	Very different answers

98

TABLE 4.16

'Salary envy' towards working groups outside General Hospital

Are there any groups on the labour market in general whose salaries are higher than yours even though their jobs are less demanding and carry less responsibility?

	Department chiefs (%)	Nurses (%)	Non-professional nursing staff (%)	Ancillary professional staff (%)	Maintenance and other staff (%)	Office staff (%)
Yes, many (3)	7	48	26	53	30	41
Yes, certain groups (2)	47	35	15	41	20	21
No, not as far as I know (1)	47	17	58	6	50	38
No. of respondents	16	121	277	17	67	31
No answer	1	9	16	0	6	2
If yes, which groups do you mean?	Completely different jobs	Completely different jobs	Completely different jobs or similar jobs with another employer	Very different answers	Very different answers	Same job but employed in private industry

99

The average values of the answers to the questions on salary were also classified according to age and employee group (see Table 4.17); again, only department chiefs were included instead of all doctors. Of the various employee groups, ancillary professional staff and nurses indicate the strongest feelings of unfair treatment and department chiefs the weakest. One explanation might be the familiar situation in which the level of aspiration becomes higher along with increased education. The department chiefs' low average values can be explained by their salary level when compared with other groups in society. Non-professional nursing staff exhibit almost the same low average values for both questions as the department chiefs. All employee groups think that they are treated much more unfairly in relation to other employee groups in General Hospital than to groups outside.

The overall picture does not change when age groups are taken into consideration, though some variations occur. With only a few exceptions, the nurses' evaluations in different age groups are above the average values for all personnel in different age groups. The opposite applies to non-professional nursing staff. The number of respondents in different age groups among the department chiefs and ancillary professional staff was too small to draw definite conclusions.

If all personnel are classified in different age groups, there seems to be some tendency for those in the lower age groups (except the lowest) to feel they are treated unfairly over salary, compared with the higher age groups. This tendency becomes even more pronounced in comparisons with employee groups on the labour market in general. But this tendency diminishes somewhat when the different age groups for each special employee category are compared. In other words, this tendency for all personnel seems somewhat illusory.

The generally critical attitude of ancillary professional staff towards these salary comparisons may arise because this group is not represented in the age groups in which other employees tend to exhibit relatively low average values. The comparatively low average values for doctors as a whole may be explained by our mistake of only including the department chiefs.

As we might expect, the two questions are closely related. Those who feel they are treated unfairly at General Hospital also think they are mistreated in comparison with the labour market in general.

100

General Hospital as a place to work compared with other places of employment

The employees were also asked to evaluate General Hospital compared with other places of employment, Industry Town compared with other areas, work supervision at General Hospital compared with their ideas of how other institutions and businesses were run, and working conditions in their own unit (clinical department or equivalent) compared with conditions in other units at General Hospital. The most striking outcome of this series of questions is the neutral and cautious nature of the answers given. Nearly half the respondents in almost all departments and professional groups evaluated General Hospital, Industry Town, and the management at General Hospital as 'about average'. The only question which evoked more decisive opinions was that comparing one's own department with other units at General Hospital. These attitudes were in favour of the employee's own department. Tables 4.18a to d show the average values for these categories according to job and age groups.

General Hospital as a place to work (Table 4.18a) was evaluated as somewhat better than average (average value = 3.2). Ancillary professional staff (3.4) and doctors (3.3) recorded a somewhat higher average value and nurses (3.0) a somewhat lower average value than other groups (3.2), though these differences are insignificant. Controls on the influence of age differences tend to indicate that the nurses' slightly lower average values can be explained by the fact that they are somewhat more critical in the younger age groups. The doctors' average value might have been higher because the department chiefs—primarily those over 50 years of age—are relatively positive towards General Hospital as a place of employment. When the various employee groups are compared on the basis of a particular age group, it emerges that ancillary professional staff are the most positive in attitude towards their place of work. The average value for all personnel is slightly lower in the age group 21 to 30 than in all other age groups. The highest age groups exhibit more positive evaluations than all other age groups. This is a familiar pattern in most attitude studies of this kind.

Industry Town as a place to live as compared with other areas

The total average value (3.0) corresponds with 'about average' on the measurement scale. In this instance, employees with academic degrees—doctors (2.8), registered nurses (2.8), and ancillary professional staff

101

TABLE 4.17

'Salary envy' towards groups within and outside General Hospital, according to age and job categories.

Average values of answers to the question: Are there groups of employees at General Hospital whose salaries are higher than yours even though their jobs are less demanding and carry less responsibility?

Age group	Personnel group						
	Department chiefs	Nurses	Non-professional nursing staff	Ancillary professional staff	Maintenance and other staff	Office staff	All staff
< 21 years	—	—	1.2	—	1.0	1.4	1.3
21-25 years	—	1.8	1.3	(1.3)	(2.0)	1.4	1.5
26-30 years	—	1.6	1.1	(1.8)	(1.5)	(1.0)	1.5
31-40 years	(2.0)	1.3	1.3	1.8	1.1	1.5	1.4
41-50 years	1.4	1.6	1.3	(2.0)	1.4	1.6	1.4
51-60 years	1.0	1.6	1.2	—	1.3	1.2	1.3
> 60 years	(1.0)	(1.3)	(1.0)	—	1.0	(1.5)	1.1
All ages	1.2	1.6	1.2	1.8	1.3	1.4	1.4
No. of respondents	16	121	277	17	67	31	529
No answer	0	12	21	0	3	4	40

Response alternatives: Yes, many groups (3), Yes, certain groups (2) and No, not as far as I know (1).

Parentheses indicate that the value could not be taken into account because the sample was too small (< 5 respondents).

Average values of answers to the question: Are there groups on the labour market in general whose salaries are higher than yours even though their jobs are less demanding and carry less responsibility?

Age group	Personnel group						
	Department chiefs	Nurses	Non-professional nursing staff	Ancillary professional staff	Maintenance and other staff	Office staff	All staff
< 21 years	–	–	1.4	–	(2.0)	1.2	1.4
21-25 years	–	2.6	2.0	(2.3)	(2.0)	2.0	2.2
26-30 years	–	2.4	1.4	(2.0)	(2.5)	(2.0)	2.1
31-40 years	(2.0)	2.2	1.8	2.7	1.8	(2.7)	2.0
41-50 years	2.0	2.3	2.0	(2.0)	1.8	2.0	2.0
51-60 years	1.4	2.3	1.4	–	1.7	1.6	1.6
> 60 years	(1.0)	(1.7)	(2.0)	–	(1.3)	1.7	1.5
All ages	1.6	2.3	1.7	2.5	1.8	1.8	1.9
No. of respondents	16	121	277	17	67	31	529
No answer	1	9	16	0	6	2	34

(2.0)–seem more critical than other employee groups–maintenance staff (3.2), other nursing staff (3.1) and office staff (3.1). The same is true in respect to the age composition of employee groups (with the exception of ancillary professional staff). But generally, in all personnel groups, employees over 40 are somewhat more positive towards Industry Town as a place to live than are other age groups.

Work supervision at General Hospital compared with other places of employment

Comparison of work supervision at General Hospital and other places of employment (Table 4.18c) showed that it is 'about average' (3.1) for all personnel. It is interesting to note that the average values for doctors (2.9) and nurses (2.8) indicate that some employees in these categories are less satisfied with the way in which work is supervised than others (3.1-3.2).

Working conditions in the employee's own unit as compared with other units at General Hospital

Less neutral results are obtained when working conditions in the employee's own department (or equivalent) are compared with those in other departments at General Hospital (Table 4.18d). The total evaluation is slightly above average (3.4). The average values for non-professional nursing personnel (3.6) and office staff (3.5) are slightly higher than those for other categories (3.3-3.4). This also seems to apply to non-professional nursing staff in all age groups. Doctors tend with increasing age to be more critical of their own departments–they are most critical in the age groups 51 to 60 years (department chiefs)–while nurses have the opposite tendency. Non-professional nursing staff are most positive in the three lowest age groups, and office staff in the lowest age group. But the most critical group comprises office staff between 21 to 25 years of age. In all personnel groups, employees are most positive in the lowest and highest age groups (3.7) and most critical between 31 and 40 years of age (3.3).

Thus, attitudes towards one's own department are fairly similar in the different professional groups. But the differences are greater between departments. The way in which the departments were assessed on the basis of the employees' evaluations more or less coincides with the way in which the hospital management assessed the various departments.

104

Members of the board were asked the same question as the personnel, i.e. to evaluate working conditions within the clinical departments. Answers in this instance centred around the standard of facilities at the disposal of the various departments, and the number of vacancies. A department with modern facilities and no personnel vacancies was ranked first, and one with outdated facilities and a large number of vacancies or temporary staff was placed far down on the list.

We also tried to make a simple evaluation of the extent to which conditions in the departments varied. We calculated coefficients of correlation for the following variables in comparisons of different departments:

Satisfaction with General Hospital as a place of employment.
Satisfaction with Industry Town as a place to live.
Satisfaction with work supervision at General Hospital.
Work supervisors' interest in personnel welfare.
Satisfaction with one's own salary scale compared with that of other groups at the hospital and other groups in society.
Length of employment at General Hospital.
Size of department (number of employees).
Degree of self-sufficiency (the less a department depends on services from outside—measured in terms of cost allocation—the higher its degree of self-sufficiency).

Most of these variables were estimated on the basis of the average values of the variables for each department. A few of these variables were obtained from personnel statistics and cost-accounting records at the hospital.

Since this study is limited to General Hospital it does not seem meaningful to try to establish significant correlations between different variables. Thus, coefficients of correlation should only be regarded as a means of describing conditions at General Hospital.

The coefficients of correlation obtained (r) are generally low $(-0.4 < r < 0.4)$. Department size is negatively correlated with satisfaction attained from working conditions in the department $(r = -0.50)$ and with supervisors' interest in personnel welfare $(r = -0.45)$. A department's degree of self-sufficiency is negatively correlated with supervisors' interest in personnel welfare $(r = -0.45)$, positively correlated with the average length of employment at General Hospital $(r = 0.77)$ and with satisfaction derived from Industry Town $(r = 0.67)$. Satisfaction with General Hospital as a place of employment is positively correlated with almost all the other variables.

105

TABLE 4.18a

General Hospital as a place of work as compared with other places of employment

Average values of answers to the question: Compared with other hospitals I think General Hospital as a place of employment is . . . (response alternatives below)

Age group	Personnel group						
	Doctors	Nurses	Non-professional nursing staff	Ancillary professional staff	Maintenance and other staff	Office staff	All personnel
< 21 years	–	–	3.2	–	(3.0)	(3.0)	3.2
21-25 years	(3.8)	2.9	3.1	(3.3)	(3.0)	(2.8)	3.1
26-30 years	3.1	2.9	3.1	(3.3)	(3.3)	(4.0)	3.0
31-40 years	3.0	3.1	3.3	3.4	3.0	(3.0)	3.2
41-50 years	3.2	3.1	3.2	(3.7)	3.2	3.1	3.2
51-60 years	4.2	3.2	3.3	–	3.3	3.4	3.3
> 60 years	(3.7)	(4.3)	(3.0)	–	(3.0)	(3.8)	3.6
All ages	3.3	3.0	3.2	3.4	3.2	3.2	3.2
No. of respondents	54	121	277	17	67	31	567
No answer	2	10	36	0	12	3	63

Response alternatives: Definitely better than average (5), Better than average (4), About average (3), Worse than average (2), Definitely worse than average (1).

Parentheses indicate that the value could not be taken into account because the sample was too small (< 5 respondents).

106

TABLE 4.18b

Industry Town as a place to live as compared with other areas

Average values of answers to the question: Compared with other areas where I could be living, Industry Town as a place to live is . . . (response alternatives given opposite)

Age group	Personnel group						
	Doctors	Nurses	Non-professional nursing staff	Ancillary professional staff	Maintenance and other staff	Office staff	All personnel
< 21 years	—	—	3.0	—	(3.0)	3.0	3.0
21-25 years	(2.0)	2.7	3.2	(3.3)	(3.3)	3.0	3.0
26-30 years	2.8	2.6	3.0	(2.5)	(3.3)	(2.0)	2.8
31-40 years	2.7	2.8	3.1	3.0	3.0	(3.7)	3.0
41-50 years	2.9	2.9	3.2	(2.8)	3.1	3.1	3.1
51-60 years	3.3	3.1	3.2	—	3.3	3.2	3.2
> 60 years	(3.0)	(3.0)	(3.0)	—	(3.3)	(3.0)	3.1
All ages	2.8	2.8	3.1	2.9	3.2	3.1	3.0
No. of respondents	54	121	277	17	67	31	567
No answer	2	2	12	0	6	0	22

TABLE 4.18c

Work supervision at General Hospital as compared with other places of employment

Average values of answers to the question: Compared with other places of employment I think work supervision at General Hospital is . . . (response alternatives below)

Age group	Personnel group						
	Doctors	Nurses	Non-professional nursing staff	Ancillary professional staff	Maintenance and other staff	Office staff	All personnel
< 21 years	–	–	3.1	–	(0.5)	3.4	3.2
21-25 years	(3.0)	2.6	3.1	(3.7)	(2.7)	2.6	3.0
26-30 years	2.9	2.7	3.0	(2.8)	(3.0)	(3.0)	2.8
31-40 years	2.9	3.0	3.1	3.2	3.9	(3.0)	3.0
41-50 years	2.8	2.8	3.3	–	3.4	2.8	3.2
> 60 years	(3.0)	(4.5)	(3.0)	–	(2.5)	(3.8)	3.4
All ages	2.9	2.8	3.2	3.1	3.1	3.1	3.1
No. of respondents	54	121	277	17	67	31	567
No answer	2	11	22	0	6	1	42

Response alternatives: Definitely better than average (5), Better than average (4), About average (3), Worse than average (2), Definitely worse than average (1).

Parentheses indicate that the value could not be taken into account because the sample was too small (< 5 respondents).

108

TABLE 4.18d

Working conditions in the employee's own unit compared with other units

Average values of answers to the question: Compared with other units at General Hospital, working conditions in my unit (department or equivalent) are ... (response alternatives given opposite)

Age group	Personnel group						
	Doctors	Nurses	Non-professional nursing staff	Ancillary professional staff	Maintenance and other staff	Office staff	All personnel
< 21 years	–	–	3.6	–	(3.0)	4.0	3.7
21-25 years	3.8	3.2	3.7	(3.7)	(3.7)	2.0	3.5
26-30 years	3.4	3.2	3.9	(3.8)	(4.3)	(4.0)	3.5
31-40 years	3.4	3.1	3.4	2.8	3.1	(4.3)	3.3
41-50 years	2.7	3.5	3.5	–	3.3	3.4	3.4
> 60 years	(3.7)	(5.0)	(3.5)	–	3.0	(3.8)	3.7
All ages	3.3	3.3	3.6	3.4	3.3	3.5	3.4
No. of respondents	54	121	277	17	67	31	567
No answer	3	4	20	0	3	0	30

Staff turnover

The hospital's personnel records are so unsatisfactory that it is almost impossible to obtain accurate information on staff turnover without resorting to an extensive survey. The management consultants mentioned earlier did carry out one study covering 1963-67, and the results are shown in Table 4.19. Employment of nurses and doctors is somewhat better

TABLE 4.19

Staff turnover per department and personnel category at General Hospital[38]

Department	Staff turnover (%)	Average no. of employees
Medicine	22	92
Surgery	18	123
Obstetrics and Gynaecology	24	77
Paediatrics	18	51
Ear, nose and throat	28	32
Ophthalmology	26	18
Chest	25	19
Long-term care	N/A	N/A
Psychiatry	17	62
Radiotherapy	20	43
Infectious diseases	18	73
Central laboratory	21	42
Rehabilitation	39	6
Anaesthetics	33	8
Intensive care	32	10
Category		
Department chiefs	10	14
Other doctors	147	33
Registered nurses	24	167
Midwives	66	7
Physiotherapists	57	7
Occupational therapists	86	6
Medical secretaries	9	31
X-ray and laboratory assistants	12	29
Assistant and paediatric nurses	6	91
Non-professional nursing staff	53	336

documented, probably because recruitment in these two categories is regarded as a more serious problem. Table 4.20 reflects the situation at the end of 1965.

We asked employees how long they thought that they would continue to work at General Hospital. Answers were classified into employee and age groups according to the average values (Table 4.22). Doctors and ancillary professional staff exhibit an 'employment curve' which differs from all other groups. As far as the doctors are concerned, this might be explained by the fact that the group as a whole contains four subgroups with varying employment behaviour (locums who remain only a few months, junior doctors with three-year appointments, assistant department chiefs, and department chiefs with permanent appointments).

The measurement scales could be criticised because the time intervals are of varying lengths. This means that conclusions cannot be drawn on the basis of the absolute size of the average values. The table serves only to illustrate the relative differences in average values between different employee and age groups. Maintenance and non-professional nursing staff in particular, and also office staff, plan to remain at General Hospital longer than other groups; doctors and ancillary professional staff, for the shortest periods. The average time of stay which nurses envisage is midway between that of all other groups. Groups with academic degrees plan, on average, to remain at General Hospital for a shorter time than groups composed of non-graduates. These differences between employee groups are maintained if the age factor is also included. The only exception is the high average value for doctors aged between 50 and 60. This is probably because all doctors in this age group are department chiefs.

The answers also indicate a relationship between age and the time for which employees plan to remain at General Hospital. In general, it seems that the older the employee, the longer he plans to stay. For obvious reasons, this does not apply to the highest age groups for whom retirement is imminent. The wide distribution of values in the various age groups for doctors might also be explained by the different types of appointments in this category—locum appointments are more common in the lower age groups, and appointments as permanent department chiefs more common in the higher age groups.

It is difficult to determine the reliability and value of these data as a prediction of future employment trends. But we think we are justified in assuming that a fairly good picture of employees' intentions was gained and that their answers give a basis for evaluating employee behaviour. The data is consistent with the information on staff turnover given in Tables 4.19 and 4.21 and with the future resignations estimated from data

TABLE 4.20

Personnel situation with regard to doctors and nurses, 1 December 1965

Department	Nurses				Physicians (DC = department chief, ADC = assistant department chief, JD= junior doctor)			
	No. of positions	Permanently employed	Locums	Vacancies	No. of positions	Permanently employed	Locums	Vacancies
Medicine	21.5	18	2.5	1	1 DC, 4 JD	4	1	
Surgery	38.5	29.5	6	3	1 DC, 1 ADC, 4 JD	4	2	
Obstetrics, Gynaecology	13.5	10.5	2	1	1 DC, 1 ADC, 3 JD	3		
Paediatrics	8.5	5.5	2.5	0.5	1 DC, 2 JD	3	2	
Ear, nose and throat	7	3.5	1	2.5	1 DC, 2 JD	3		
Ophthalmology	6	3	2	1	1 DC, 1 ADC	2		
Infectious medicine	16	5.5	2.5*	8	1 DC, 1 ADC, 2 JD	1		
Chest	8	4.75	2.5	0.75	1 DC, 1 ADC, 1 JD	3	1	2
Orthopaedics	9	5		4	1 DC, 1 ADC, 1 JD	3		
Long-term care	26	13.5	3	9.5	1 DC, 3 JD	3		
Psychiatry	16	9.5	1	5.5	1 DC, 1 ADC, 3 JD	2		1
X-ray	12	8	4		1 DC, 1 ADC, 4 JD	4	2	1
Rehabilitation	1	1			1 DC, 1 JD	2	2	

112

Table 4.20 (continued)

Laboratory + blood bank	13	9	$4^\dagger$		1 DC, 1 JD	1	1
Anaesthetics					1 DC, 1 JD	1	1
Shared	6.5	4	2.5		55	39	11
Total	202.5	126.25	37	39.25	55	39	11	5

* 1.5 not fully qualified † 2 not qualified

concerning the length of employment for newly hired staff (Table 4.23).

We also asked employees to indicate the probable reasons why they would leave General Hospital (see Table 4.24). These results can be compared with those in Table 4.25, which gives the reasons specified by nurses for terminating their employment at General Hospital.

The hospital's unsatisfied demands

The hospital's unsatisfied demands can be measured quantitatively by the number of vacancies. This was described earlier, in connection with our study of employee's power. We tried to measure the hospital's view of the quality of the employees' contributions. We asked all supervisors to indicate how many of their subordinates they thought were suitably qualified, and how many they would like to replace if the labour market permitted more choice in recruiting. The results in Table 4.26 show that persons in supervisory positions think that all doctors and registered nurses and approximately 90 per cent of other staff fulfil their tasks satisfactorily. But if the labour market permitted, and they had complete freedom to act, supervisors would like to replace almost 25 per cent of doctors and about 10 per cent of nurses and other nursing staff.

The positive attitude of those in supervisory positions towards the contributions of their staff and particularly towards doctors and registered

TABLE 4.21

Nurse turnover, 1965

No. of nurses	Permanent	Temporary	Total
At the beginning of the year	126.25	37	163.25
Employed during the year	28	21	49
	154.25	58	212.25
Resignations during the year	28	21	49
At the end of the year	126.25	37	163.25

114

TABLE 4.22

'How long do you think you will continue to work at General Hospital?'
Average values of answers to the questions

Age group	Personnel group						
	Doctors	Nurses	Non-professional nursing staff	Ancillary professional staff	Maintenance and other staff	Office staff	All personnel
< 21 years	—	—	3.4	—	(4.0)	4.2	3.6
21-25 years	1.8	3.1	3.9	3.0	4.0	3.5	3.5
26-30 years	3.3	3.7	4.0	(3.3)	(4.3)	(4.0)	3.7
31-40 years	3.1	4.5	4.5	3.8	4.9	4.0	4.3
41-50 years	4.1	4.1	4.8	(4.0)	4.5	4.9	4.6
51-60 years	5.0	4.4	4.8	—	4.7	4.8	4.7
> 60 years	(3.7)	(3.7)	(4.5)	—	(3.5)	(4.3)	3.9
All ages	3.6	3.9	4.5	3.6	4.5	4.3	4.2
No. of respondents	54	121	277	17	61	31	567
No answer	0	4	16	0	4	2	26

Response alternatives: Less than one month (1), 1-6 months (2), 6-12 months (3), 1-3 years (4), more than 3 years (5).
Parentheses indicate that the value could not be taken into account because the sample was too small (< 5 respondents).

nurses, is consistent with the hospital management's view. Twelve people on the board and county council were asked for their opinions of the employees' contributions. Not only were their views vague, but they were also unanimously positive in their evaluations (to the extent that they dared make any). In other words, the supervisors' views imply evaluations with various shades of meaning.

TABLE 4.23

No. of employees still working at General Hospital who began between 1961-65 as compared with answers to the question: 'How long do you think you will stay?'

Year	Doctors			Nurses			Non-professional nursing staff		
	No employed at the beginning of the year	Remaining in Feb. 1966	Expected to remain until Feb. 1966	No. employed at the beginning of the year	Remaining in Feb. 1966	Expected to remain until Feb. 1966	No. employed at the beginning of the year	Remaining in Feb.1966	Expected to remain until Feb. 1966
	*	%	%	*	%	%	*	%	%
1961	41	35	33	146	46	23	319	54	54
1962	46	41	35	186	54	29	411	63	58
1963	49	46	38	175	63	35	403	70	64
1964	53	51	55	176	71	72	422	78	88
1965	58	65	65	198	85	85	499	88	93
1966	58			196			523		

* Source: General Hospital personnel statistics (annual report).

116

Ancillary professional staff			Maintenance and other staff			Office staff		
No. employed at the beginning of the year *	Remaining in Feb. 1966 %	Expected to remain until Feb. 1966 %	No. employed at the beginning of the year *	Remaining in Feb. 1966 %	Expected to remain until Feb. 1966 %	No. employed at the beginning of the year *	Remaining in Feb. 1966 %	Expected to remain until Feb. 1966 %
29	19	25	87	54	54	41	35	40
36	28	28	94	63	58	50	41	45
37	39	29	94	70	64	51	46	50
43	51	52	95	78	88	56	55	83
55	65	75	103	88	93	70	75	92
67			108			73		

TABLE 4.24

Reasons which employees gave for resigning from General Hospital

Expected reasons for terminating one's job	Doctors %	Nurses %	Non-professional nursing staff %	Ancillary professional staff %	Maintenance and other staff %	Office staff %
1 Retirement	24	24	24	12	45	26
2 Family moving away	7	19	18	12	5	7
3 Devote oneself to family	0	18	28	0	8	19
4 New job in Industry Town	0	4	7	0	17	16
5 New job in another area	44	20	9	53	12	16
6 Other reason	24	14	13	23	14	13
No. of respondents	54	119	267	17	65	31
No answer	0	2	10	0	2	0

TABLE 4.25

Nurses' reasons for terminating their employment

Those who left did so for the following reasons	Number	%
1 Moving from the area	15	31
2 Family reasons	11	22
3 Studies	6	12
4 Dissatisfied with job	2	4
5 Better pay somewhere else (in private industry)	3	6
6 Intended to work on a substitute basis only	7	14
7 Retirement	5	10
	49	100

118

TABLE 4.26

Management view of subordinate personnel[39]

	Department chiefs' evaluation of		Charge nurses' evaluation of		Other supervisors' evaluation of subordinate personnel
	Doctors	Nurses	Nurses	Non-professional nursing staff	
We supervise . . .	39	145	47	276	194
. . . of these employees have been with us long enough for us to evaluate their qualifications	30	134	47	257	157
. . . of those we think that we can evaluate are sufficiently qualified to fulfil the tasks they were employed to do	28	123	45	244	162
while . . . are insufficiently qualified	8	13	2	25	15
We feel that . . . of our subordinates exhibit the willingness to work and perform the quantity of work we think should be asked of them	37	141	46	245	175
while . . . exhibit unsatisfactory willingness to work or perform an insufficient amount of work	1	4	1	26	16
We think we can evaluate . . . with respect to willingness to work and amount of work performed	39	143	47	257	181
If there were an abundance of manpower and we could act freely we would retain . . . of these persons	29	131	45	242	171
while we would try to replace . . . by more suitable persons	9	14	2	28	15
We feel that we can evaluate . . .	37	145	47	274	181

119

Notes

[1] According to health care legislation, the county is not required to be responsible for preventive care (such as pre-natal care, child health care or chest X-ray examinations). However, since there is general agreement as to the importance of preventive medicine, all county authorities offer this kind of care as a matter of course.

[2] For a more detailed definition of the contribution-inducement balance, see chapter 2.

[3] In accordance with legislation, or as a generally accepted practice, the county council is responsible for public dental care, special institutions for handicapped children, etc.

[4] A simplified fee system known as the 'seven-crown reform' for public outpatient care took effect on 1 January, 1970. At each visit, the patient pays only part (7 cr.) of the physician's total fee. The remainder is paid directly to the county council by the National Social Insurance Service.

[5] There are no longer any private or semi-private rooms available at the hospitals in the county.

[6] See note 4.

[7] A new agreement for most of the doctors not in private practice took effect on 1 January, 1970. According to this new agreement, the previous system of salaries and compensation was replaced by a total salary; fixed working hours were also introduced, and regulations governing compensation for on-call service were changed.

[8] Salaries and other compensation for persons employed by the county council (as in other public administration) are regulated by agreements between the Association of County Councils and the employee organisations. The most important are the Swedish Municipal Workers' Union (affiliated with the Swedish Confederation of Trade Unions) which negotiates for student nurses and nursing auxiliaries, the Swedish Association of Public Health Officers (associated with the Swedish Central Organisation of Salaried Employees), which negotiates for the nurses, and the Swedish Medical Association (affiliated with the Swedish Confederation of Professional Associations), which negotiates on behalf of doctors.

Central and regional negotiations usually take place once every three years. Each county council negotiates with the employees' unions on the regional level. Two salary schemes (KB and KA), which cover a number of salary grades, apply to staff employed by the council. All personnel categories receive extra compensation for overtime and on-call and back-up service. Employees on night duty receive higher salaries than those who work during the day. For a transitional period, doctors also

120

receive additional pay on a monthly basis in order to compensate for their salary loss in connection with the new salary system which came into effect on 1 January, 1970 (see note 9).

Average monthly salaries, including additional compensation, paid to the different categories of doctors are as follows (1972):

Department chief	approx. 12,000 cr.
Assistant department chief	10-11,000 cr.
Junior doctor	9-10,000 cr.

[9] New legislation, to take effect in 1973, was passed in 1970, limiting normal working time to a maximum of 40 hours per week (excluding breaks).

[10] The Central Board of Hospital Planning and the National Council for Hospital Rationalisation were replaced in 1968 by the Institute for the Planning and Rationalisation of Health and Social Welfare Services. This Institute is run jointly by the state and the county councils.

[11] This situation made us wonder whether the study should be replanned to include the entire county council. But the resources we had at our disposal did not permit this.

[12] See notes 4 and 7.

[13] See the Swedish Government's instruction to the National Medical Board, 3 December, 1965 (no. 778).

[14] Some changes in health legislation were made in 1971. The health and medical services board was assigned the responsibility of dividing health and medical care areas into districts, and hospitals into departments and other units (or, if called for, the joining of departments into blocs). The purpose of this legislation was to give the authorities more freedom to set up the administrative organisation with regard to rationalisation and local conditions.

[15] See note 1 to chapter 6.

[16] If state subsidies are granted, the matter is decided by the Swedish Government.

[17] Direct taxes on income are paid on both a national and a county basis. Taxes paid to the state are progressive, and those paid to the county are directly proportional to income. County taxes are used partly to cover the expenses incurred by the county council. In 1973 this amount was, on average, 9.30 cr. per 100 cr. of taxable income.

[18] Assistant department chiefs are usually also members of these organisations.

[19] Our results on this point differ from those reported in B.M. Bernheim,

Story of the Johns Hopkins: Four Great Doctors and the Medical School they Created, World's Work, New York 1949; L. Freeman, *Hospital in Action: the Story of the Michael Reese Medical Center*, Rand McNally, Chicago 1956; and T. Burling, E. M. Lents, and R. N. Wilson (eds.), *The Give and Take in Hospitals*, New York 1956. These studies indicate that medical and surgical department chiefs often have major positions in a hospital. The absence of this situation in our report may be caused by the previously mentioned periods of absence of some department chiefs while our study was in progress (see chapter 3).

[20] This conclusion is based on statements made by department chiefs, the hospital board of trustees and county council representatives. See our evaluations later in chapter 4, after having studied actual decision-making. C. Perrow reports on similar conditions at American hospitals in *Authority, Goals and Prestige in a General Hospital* (unpublished doctoral dissertation) University of California, Berkeley 1960; and in 'Goals and Power Structure—Historical Case Study' in E. Freidson (ed.), *Hospital in Modern Society*, The Free Press of Glencoe, New York 1963.

[21] There is also agreement between answers to the question 'how easy would it be for you to obtain another job?' and 'how attractive do you think these other jobs are?'

[22] Junior doctors are not completely in agreement on this issue.

[23] We base this assumption solely on informal observations and statements.

[24] Decisions were made in 1969 regarding a new system for the further education of doctors. According to these decisions, basic medical school education, which lasts five and a half years, is to be followed by 21 months' obligatory internship. This is to be followed by specialisation, after which the doctor is declared competent as a specialist in a particular field of medicine.

A new scheme for doctors will take effect in 1973. During their period of internship and general or specialist education, they will serve in the capacity of junior doctors. The hospital will have positions available for doctors who have completed their education as ward doctors, assistant department chiefs, or department chiefs. With respect to outpatient care outside the hospital, there will be positions for district medical officers and assistant district medical officers in the various regions. These positions will be filled by general practitioners, as well as specialists.

[25] It is difficult to estimate the exact sum under negotiation because the demands involved are not always expressed in crowns.

[26] Gränges AB (the Grängesberg Company) is a large Swedish firm with 26,000 employees, and annual sales amounting to three billion crowns.

[27] See note 4.

[28] One of the main aims of the 'seven-crown reform' (see note 4 above) was to equalise the economic burden on in-patients and outpatients, and as a result, to reduce the pressure on in-patient care and thus facilitate expansion of outpatient care.

[29] However, the number of complaints registered with the National Board of Health and Welfare has increased considerably during the last few years.

[30] The political status of members of the hospital board was measured on the basis of the votes cast for the various political parties in the county council election of 1963, the local election of 1962, and the Parliamentary elections of 1964.

A status scale from 0 to 10 was constructed. Ten meant that a representative was placed in the upper tenth of a ballot for all three elections. Zero meant that the name did not appear on any ballot. Figure 4.6 shows that, with two exceptions, all members had relatively low status figures. This relates to the fact that their names only appeared on one ballot (local or county council elections). None of the members of the hospital board was on the ballot list for the 1964 parliamentary elections.

[31] KB1 = 63080 cr. in 1973.

[32] See note 4.

[33] Income includes compensation for in-patient and outpatient care. Total annual incomes were estimated for doctors employed for less than one year. Radiologists and pathologists are excluded because their income does not depend on the number of hours of outpatient care.

[34] Some examples of ways in which the department chiefs identified with the personnel against their employer are as follows. One physician said that he had advised a junior doctor not to accept a job in his department in order to force the county council to raise the salary for this position. Several chiefs had been in conflict with the personnel department or management in an attempt to obtain higher salaries for medical secretaries.

When the National Board of Health and Welfare asked the board at General Hospital to reduce the number of junior doctors employed during the summer, the department chiefs did not support this request. Instead, they sided with the junior doctors who wanted a decrease in their workload (possible so long as the number of appointments was not reduced). Many department chiefs are highly sceptical towards rationalising food service at the hospital because it would involve lowering nutritional standards for the patients.

[35] See note 9.

123

[36] The hospital has become increasingly dependent on the municipal housing authorities since its own allotment of housing for personnel has remained almost constant for more than fifteen years.

[37] During the most recent (1971) negotiations between the Association of County Councils and various employee unions, a decision was made whereby members on the lowest salary level (up to KA13) would receive an overall increase in salary. Thus, the differences between various categories of medical personnel are gradually being reduced.

[38] As can be seen from the table, turnover is at almost the same level for all departments: 2-30 per cent. The high values for rehabilitation, anaesthetics and intensive care may be explained by the considerably smaller number of employees in these departments.

[39] These questions were not answered by the nursing supervisors.

124

5 The Hospital's Production System

The hospital is an organisation which has many participants, all of whom depend on it to satisfy certain demands. This chapter describes activities within the hospital which are aimed at satisfying the participant group designated as the hospital's 'customers'. These activities will be termed the hospital's 'production system'. (Chapter 2 indicated some reasons for including this description in a study based on a business administration approach.) The hospital's products, production methods, and production system determine to a large extent the demands which have to be met by the hospital's administration.

In studying production within the hospital, we begin by examining the hospital's products in the light of the demands of the hospital's customers described in the preceding chapter. We then describe the productive com-

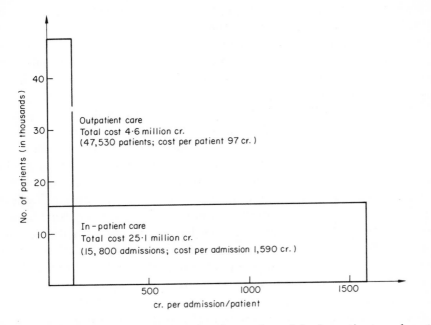

Fig. 5.1 Comparison of the 'production volume' in in-patient and out-patient care.[1]

125

ponents, and analyse the work in the various subsystems (clinical departments) which comprise the hospital.[2]

As in chapter 4, many of our results are recorded in diagrams and tables. In interpreting them, we emphasise noteworthy findings. Sometimes, comparisons are made with other organisations such as industrial firms. In some instances, we have collected information about past and present changes in the hospital's production. We conclude this chapter by summarising the main features of production at the hospital. The demands which production places on the administration are discussed in chapters 6 and 7. But the experienced reader will certainly be able to use the description in this chapter to draw his own conclusions about the distinctive demands that have to be satisfied by the administration of such a unique production system as a hospital.

The hospital's products

Primary and secondary products

The hospital has two primary products: outpatient and in-patient care. More patients are cared for as outpatients, but in-patient care costs more. The hospital also produces certain secondary products such as medical check-ups, research, physiotherapy, education (for student nurses and junior doctors), and different kinds of services to other health care institutions, insurance companies, etc.

Somewhat less than half the doctors have research projects in progress (often more or less as hobbies). The hospital's educational efforts are considerable, and apply primarily to nurses. Health certificates for insurance agencies and other authorities comprise another important secondary product. It is difficult to estimate reliable production costs for writing these certificates without performing time and motion studies on the doctors. But detailed interviews did provide the estimate that between one and two full-time doctors are needed just to write certificates. Most doctors also think that demands for this 'secondary product' are increasing considerably every year. Costs of secondary products are included in the costs for in-patient and outpatient care.

It is not easy to find reliable and meaningful methods of measuring actual medical care compared with the hospital's secondary products. Our estimates show that the production costs for secondary products amount to less than 1 per cent of the hospital's total costs.

126

TABLE 5.1

General Hospital's 'products'

Products	Quantity of production	Comment
In-patient care	234,000 patient days 15,800 patients	Including outpatient X-ray examinations and physiotherapy
Outpatient care	116,000 visits 47,600 patients	
Research	40 projects	
Education	1,400 teaching hours	Mainly at the School of Nursing
Health certificates	approx. 5,000 minor 1,000 general 800 major 3,000 unclas- sified (Receipt for physician's fee excluded)	Physician's time consumed (average in each class: 10,15, 30 and 20 minutes)

Complexity of products

The complexity of a product refers to the number of steps or processes involved in 'making' it. The hospital has no statistics which directly reflect complexity. This meant that our evaluations had to be made on the basis of the hospital's own accounting information and from interviews with department chiefs.

The cost per outpatient visit varies considerably from one department to the next (see Table 5.2a). The average direct cost per patient in the long-term-care outpatient department is more than twenty times as high as the average direct cost per patient in the ophthalmology clinic. If the total cost per patient in the long-term care and ophthalmology clinics are compared, the cost in the former is only about eight times higher than the latter clinic. There are two ways of explaining these large differences. First, the long-term-care clinic receives a very small share of total outpatient visits (less than 1 per cent) so that fixed costs are distributed over a smaller base. Second, according to the doctors, the figures also reflect differences in the complexity of the product, if complexity is defined as the number of treatment steps.

Table 5.2a also shows that the rehabilitation clinic accounts for the largest number of visits per patient (6) while the ophthalmology, paediatric, and gynaecology clinics have the lowest number (1.5 and 1.7, respectively). The surgical and long-term care clinics are in the middle of the scale with 2.8 and 3.3 visits per patient, respectively. The cost per visit varies considerably: 28 cr. in the surgical clinic, 140 cr. in the long-term care clinic.

The picture is somewhat different with respect to in-patient care (see Table 5.2b). The differences in the cost per patient and the average length of stay are still large, but less so than for outpatient care. This also corresponds with the way in which different departments describe treatment of 'typical patients'. However, comparisons between different departments are not sufficient to understand the difference between the most and least complicated cases. It is impossible to determine the cost of extreme cases unless the variations within a single department are studied.

TABLE 5.2a

Volume and cost of care in clinical departments: outpatients.

Clinical department	Volume of care			Cost per patient		Cost per visit	
	No. of patients (in thousands)	No. of visits	Visits per patient	Direct costs (cr.)	Direct + indirect costs (cr.)	Direct costs (cr.)	Direct + indirect costs (cr.)
Medicine	3.9	11.6	3.0	75	150	25	50
Surgery	10.2	36.1	3.3	41	92	12	28
Obstetrics and Gynaecology	5.6	9.7	1.7	31	52	18	30
Paediatric	3.0	4.6	1.5	34	49	23	33
Ear, nose and throat	6.3	19.2	3.0	16	71	5	23
Ophthalmology	6.3	9.7	1.5	9	48	6	31
Infectious diseases	0.7	2.2	3.1	113	187	37	60
Orthopaedics	2.3	4.3	1.9	65	108	35	58
Long-term care	0.4	1.1	2.8	209	378	77	140
Psychiatry	0.7	2.1	3.0	196	325	72	120
Child psychiatry	0.02	0.04	2.0	1,368	1,554	934	1,061
Rehabilitation	0.2	1.2	6.0	411	879	73	156
Entire hospital	47.2	101.8	2.2	39	96	15	39

128

TABLE 5.2b

Volume and cost of care in clinical department: in-patients.

Clinical department	Volume of care			Cost per day		Cost per patient	
	No, of patient days (in thousands)	No. of patients	Average length of stay in days	Direct costs (cr.)	Direct + indirect costs (cr.)	Direct costs (cr.)	Direct + indirect costs (cr.)
Medicine	35.1	2.4	15.0	46	113	582	1,659
Surgery	34.6	2.8	12.4	39	123	481	1,520
Obstetrics and Gynaecology	12.4	2.0	6.2	48	132	288	787
Paediatries	14.8	1,8	8.2	64	117	527	578
Ear, nose and throat	8.5	1,3	6.5	47	117	314	955
Ophthalmology	5.4	0.4	13.5	55	109	802	1,598
Infectious diseases	16.6	1.6	10.4	78	142	797	1,449
Orthopaedics	7.3	0.5	14.6	34	103	449	1,369
Long-term care	58.6	0.3	195.3	34	68	6,521	2,895
Psychiatry	8.7	0.3	29.0	80	139	2,541	4,405
Rehabilitation	3.9	0.2	19.5	30	94	635	2,026
Chest	14.6	0.5	29.2	49	125	1,507	3,832
Entire hospital	220.5	14.1	359.8	48	107	708	1,591

Costs of about 100,000 cr. per patient are not unusual for emergencies and long hospital stays. Other departments also have their share of highly complicated cases. An example of the treatment administered and the costs for a case of long duration is shown in Table 5.3. Cases of short duration and few treatment measures include appendectomies and varicotomies.

Figures 5.2a, 5.2b, 5.3a, and 5.3b are flowcharts which illustrate the differences in the complexity of cases. The course of treatment for typical patients in the ear, nose and throat and medical clinics, as well as the department of surgery, is shown.

Range and distribution of assortment

We use the term 'assortment' to refer to the different types of treatment and care available at the hospital. We can get some idea of this assortment

129

TABLE 5.3

A complicated case can require hundreds of steps and cost thousands of crowns

	cr.
Bed, 100 days at 200 cr. per day	20,000
Albumin at 213 cr. per 100 ml	12,450
Blood	910
8 X-ray examinations at 20 cr. each	160
2 electrophoresis examinations	20
Doktacilin	645
Gamma globulin	240
Actocortin	400
Intravenous solutions (glucose, fats)	930
Patch tests, 100 days at 25 cr.	2,500
7 operations (average time per operation, 2 hours)	2,965
Total	41,120

by learning about the various departments within the hospital and the resources at their disposal. One measurement of the range of assortment is the number of diagnoses classified in each department. This can be obtained from the hospital's diagnosis statistics which are based on the National Board of Health and Welfare's classification of diagnoses and treatment for in-patients (an extended version of the ICDA coding of diagnoses). Table 5.4a shows that most departments treat several hundred diagnoses. But considerably fewer categories of diagnoses are cared for in the orthopaedic, X-ray, rehabilitation, and ophthalmology departments. These statistics refer in principle to the primary diagnosis for each patient. Sometimes, however, a patient might have several diagnoses, as can be seen by comparing the number of diagnoses with the number of admissions, for example, in the departments of medicine, long-term care, and infectious medicine.

Patients who are hospitalised are classified according to diagnosis. Depending on the specialty, there may be a large number of patients in each of a few diagnosis categories, e.g. in the obstetrics and gynaecology, ear, nose and throat, and surgical departments. On the other hand, there may be relatively few patients in each diagnosis classification, but a larger number of categories, e.g. in the long-term care, infectious medicine, and rehabilitation departments.

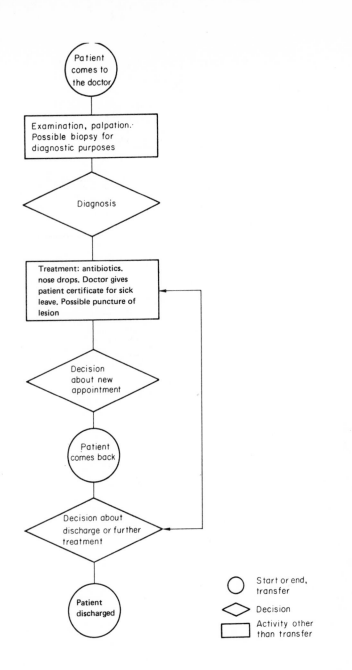

Fig. 5.2a Course of treatment in ear, nose, and throat clinic for a patient with an acute upper respiratory infection (product with a low degree of complexity).

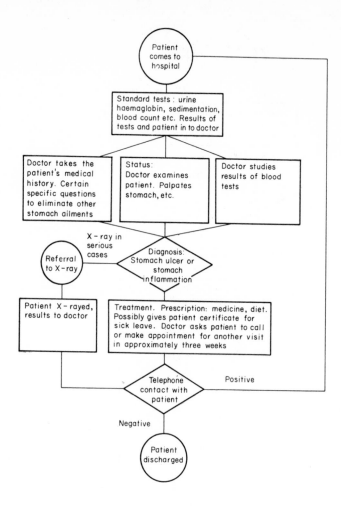

Fig. 5.2b Course of treatment in the medical clinic for patient with (non-bleeding) stomach ulcer (product with a normal degree of complexity).

132

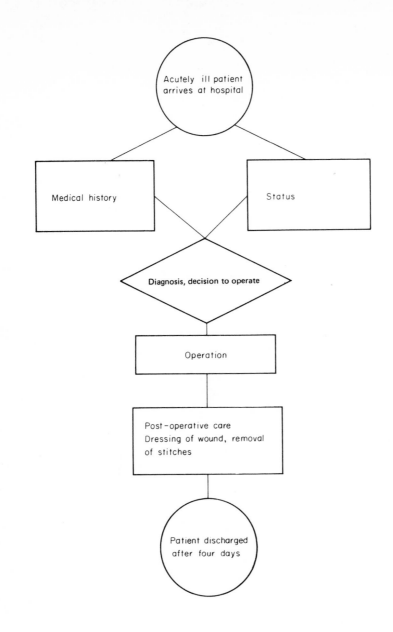

Fig. 5.3a Course of treatment in the in-patient surgical department for patient with acute appendicitis (product with a low degree of complexity).

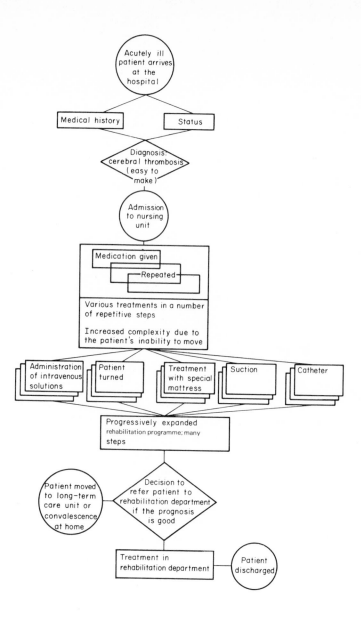

Fig. 5.3b Course of treatment in the department of medicine for patient with thrombosis (product with a high degree of complexity).

The number of diagnoses classified according to the most common diagnosis codes is a measurement of the distribution of assortment. According to column 8 in Table 5.4a, the range in the number of diagnoses, expressed as a percentage of admissions, is very large (from 6 to 34 per cent). Between 10 and 20 per cent of the patients admitted to most of the departments are classified under the departments' most common diagnosis code.

Diagnosis generally results in treatment. Another measure of the treatment assortment can be illustrated by the statistics on operations carried out in those departments where surgery is performed. In this context, we can disregard the following departments: chest clinic (whose operations are performed by other departments), infectious medicine (where very few operations are performed), and orthopaedics (which was not established until 1965). Table 5.4b shows that, of more than 5,000 operations performed annually at the hospital, the surgery and gynaecology departments show the greatest variety with an average of only four operations per operation code number. This is followed by the ear, nose and throat and ophthalmology departments. The importance of specialisation becomes apparent if we study column 2 of the table. Nearly 500 operation code numbers are used by the department of surgery, and 24 by the ophthalmology department. If combinations of diagnoses and therapeutic measures are also taken into account, the assortment is almost as large as the number of patients.

There are three different levels of care provided at the hospital: intensive, normal, and light. Some of the differences between these levels of care are shown in Table 5.5. (Note that patients often receive several levels of care during their stay at the hospital.)

When we discussed the assortment of treatments with people at the hospital, they maintained that every statistic based on types of illnesses or treatment is misleading. They felt that 'production' within a hospital is, and has to be, characterised by the fact that it should not be standardised. Each individual case is, and should be, treated as unique. To some extent, this does not only apply in a hospital but also in many industrial firms and other organisations. Even if firms classify their products in an attempt to standardise various phases of production, a certain amount of adaptation to the individual customer has to occur. The hospital's situation is probably unique in this respect. Even so, we did not feel the extent of standardisation or adaptation could be measured systematically.

135

TABLE 5.4a

Admissions, no. of diagnoses, and diagnosis numbers in twelve departments

Clinical department	Admissions	No. of diagnoses	Diagnoses per patient admitted (2) : (1)	No. of diagnosis codes
	(1)	(2)	(3)	(4)
Medicine	2,385	4,575*	2	355
Surgery	2,805	3,337*	1.2	284
Obstetrics and gynaecology	4,139	4,668	1.3	329
Paediatrics	1,813	2,335	1.2	433
Ear, nose and throat	1,284	1,479*	1.1	128
Ophthalmology	372	512	1.4	54
Chest clinic	477	303*	0.6	108
Long-term care	309	1,059	3.4	251
Orthopaedics	548	475	0.9	112
Radiotherapy	180	102	0.9	44
Rehabilitation	65	285	1.6	156
Infectious diseases	1,619	2,231	1.4	431
	16,048†	21,467	1.3	2,685

* This figure refers to patients discharged during the year.
† Patients in some departments are discharged for the weekend and readmitted on Monday, so this figure provides a somewhat erroneous picture.

Source: Annual report of the hospital, 1965.

136

Patients admitted per diagnosis code	Most common diagnosis code		No. of diagnoses for the most common diagnosis code	(7) as % of (1)
(5)	(6)		(7)	(8)
6.7	420	Morbus arteriosceleroti-cus cordis	701	29
9.9	584	Cholelithiasis	439	16
11.3	680	Partus normalis complica-tion non indicata	1,141	28
4.2	793.69	Observationes casus abdominis UNS	121	6
10.0	510	Tons.chron. ectomia non indicata	431	34
6.9	387.01	Glaucoma simplex	75	20
4.4	241	Asthma bronch.	70	15
1.2	420	Morbus arterioscleroticus cordis	69	22
4.9	735.21	Morbi cartilaginum inter-vertebralium lumbalium cum prolapsu disci	52	9
2.7	170.91	Neopl.malign.mammae	16	25
1.2	332.19	Thrombosis cerebri alia s UNS	13	7
3.8	050.99	Scarlatina alia s UNS	160	10
6			3,288	20

Demands on the quality of products

Demands on the quality of the products are made from several different quarters. Patients present their demands to the physician directly, via different participants who assume responsibility for protecting the patients' interest (primarily the National Board of Health and Welfare, the county council, and the press). Quality norms are also formulated in the doctors' basic education and subsequent practical training. We have heard doctors discuss this among themselves, and explain to one another what is meant by accepted medical practice. This latter type of quality surveillance originates within the professional group; the patient and other participants seem only to have an indirect influence.

The patients' demands with respect to quality are aimed primarily at the doctor and can be divided into two main aspects:

1 Demands on technical behaviour, i.e. on the technique of examination and treatment.
2 Demands on emotional behaviour, i.e. how the physician conducts himself. Patients believe that they should be received in a friendly manner, that the doctor should devote a certain amount time to them, listen to their problems, etc.

In addition, the patient makes demands on the hospital for adequate service, short waiting times, etc.

Successful treatment in many instances depends on whether the doctor is able to apply a suitable combination of technical and emotional behaviour. On the other hand, certain types of illnesses such as appendectomies or broken legs are linked with significant demands on technical behaviour. Outpatients sometimes express their demands for quality by visiting another doctor or departments.[3] This often applies to patients with symptoms that cannot be diagnosed as a specific illness. By changing doctors, the patient shows that he or she is dissatisfied with the first doctor's opinion. This often leads to repetition of examinations which have already been performed.

Demands on quality made by legislators and the National Board of Health and Welfare are evident in the laws, recommendations, and instructions issued to the hospital. It is important to distinguish between demands which can be carried out, and those which are only formulated as requests from the participants. Demands which, if not met, lead to actions from legislators or the board can be measured on the basis of statistics on lawsuits and disciplinary measures.

138

A review of the cases handled in 1964 by the disciplinary committee of the National Board of Health and Welfare shows that less than 10 per cent led to warnings or reprimands. About 50 per cent of the cases concern complaints that receipts, health certificates, referrals, etc. were not written out by the doctor, or that the patient was not courteously received at the hospital. Most reports concern doctors in private practice. Some of the reports are probably based on unsatisfactory medical results. But all cases in which doctors were considered to be at fault were those in which the doctors in question had used unaccepted methods of treatment. The difficulty in measuring and evaluating the quality of medical care stems from the fact that standards for the quality of the products are hardly ever formulated. Instead, standards are set with respect to methods of treatment and care. They refer to procedures and processes, but not results.

Delivery time

Delivery time is defined as the time elapsing from the moment the patient requests care until he receives it at the hospital. Measurement of an acceptable length of delivery time is difficult because urgency is evaluated in different ways by people with highly varying bases for evaluation. First, the patient has to have become aware of his need for treatment or care through his own observation of symptoms, visits to a doctor outside the hospital, or in some other way. He might come to the hospital to obtain a medical certificate. The patient can choose between three ways of making his needs known, i.e. by referral from a doctor outside the hospital, by making an appointment at an outpatient clinic, or by requesting the doctor on call for immediate care. We interviewed patients to find out how this decision was made and to determine whether their choice is based on evaluations of the length of delivery time.

In general, if a patient comes to the emergency-room, his greatest demand is for immediate help, while making an appointment means that he is willing to wait his turn. Most patients come to the hospital after having made appointments at an outpatient clinic (in all departments except one). There are no statistics on the number of emergencies and referrals so that comparisons of different departments could not be made.

When making appointments, patients do not usually have direct contact with a physician. They talk to a secretary or reception nurse on the telephone. We studied this patient-secretary contact in detail. We assumed that every patient could be classified by the number of days he indicated

139

as a 'desirable delivery time' and instructed the secretary to say: 'Yes, that would be all right .... When would you like to come?' We soon found that a numerical scale could not be used to code the answers. First, the patients' ideas were extremely vague. Common answers to the secretary's question were:'As soon as possible.' 'I don't know—sometime soon.' 'Put me in line.' The patients were often surprised by the question itself, and said: 'You have a waiting list, don't you?' It turned out that most of the patients did not make demands for quick treatment, and were prepared to wait a fairly long time.

TABLE 5.4b

Operations in the six departments where surgery is performed, 1964

Clinical department	No. of operations	No. of codes for operations	No. of operations per operation code number (1) : (2)
	(1)	(2)	(3)
Surgery	2,018	481	4.2
Obstetrics and gynaecology	1,829	431	4.2
Ear, nose and throat	939	167	5.6
Ophthalmology	183	24	7.6
Chest*	332	22	15.0
Orthopaedics	388	202	1.9
Infectious diseases	17	9	1.9
	5,706	1,336	4.3

* Statistics for the chest clinic indicate 332 operations performed on 153 patients. Figures for other departments usually refer to one operation per patient.
Some of the chest clinic's operations were performed at another hospital.
† The appendix is often removed during a number of operations and is not the main reason for the operation.

Source: Annual report of the hospital, 1965.

140

Second, the patients fall into two groups with respect to their demands on the length of delivery time, i.e. 'acutely', or 'not acutely ill' (as described in the hospital's own terms). We might include a third group comprising those who made definite requests to come at a specific time, though this was not determined by the nature of their illness but by other reasons such as working hours, free time, etc. (see Fig. 5.4).

Important differences were also observed between departments which we studied only by conducting interviews. Patients who call to make appointments are usually willing to be put on the waiting list. 'Acutely ill'

Most common operation	No. of cases for the most common operation codes	(5) as % of (1)
(4)	(5)	(6)
5,350 Cholecystectomi + draining	359	17.8
4,510 Appendectomi en passant † and inversiv app.	194	10.6
2,710 Tonsillectomia bilat.	252	26.8
1,722 Extractio combinata intracapsularis	44	24.0
Thorakocentes (ev + intreapleural treatment)	168	50.6
0,361 Exstirpation morbi cartilaginum intervertebralium alii s UNS	50	12.9
Incision	4	23.5
	1,071	18.8

TABLE 5.5

Levels of care at General Hospital[4]

Level of care	Equipment	Personnel	Surveillance
Intensive care (12 beds)	3 respirators 2 pulmotors Defibrillator ECG Cardioverter Oscilloscope Electric pulse counter Electric thermometer Electric suction apparatus Cooling mattresses Antidecubitus mattresses Rotating bed + standard equipment for a normal care unit	Day: 3-4 registered nurses, 2 assistant nurses. Night: 2 registered nurses, 1 assistant nurse or auxiliary.	Constant surveillance of patient by nurse or auxiliary. Doctors make rounds at least twice a day.
Normal care (44 departments with approx. 20 beds each)	Medicine cabinet Instrument cabinet Large autoclave Treatment carts Stretchers ECG (Medicine) Suction apparatus Oxygen Ruben's bag	Day: 1-2 registered nurses, 4-5 auxiliary. Night: 1 night nurse shared by two units, and 1 auxiliary. Extra bedside attendant if needed.	Patient can ring for auxiliary or nurse. Doctor or nurse makes rounds about five times a day (extra bedside attendant available for constant surveillance if needed).
Light care (32 beds)	Pantry	1 assistant nurse. Unit closed on weekends.	Patient should be able to take care of his own hygiene.

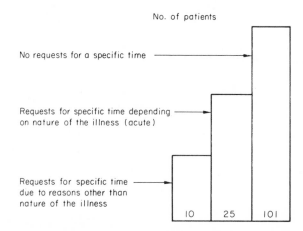

Fig. 5.4   Patients' expressed wishes as to length of delivery time (department of ophthalmology).

142

patients come directly to the hospital, or call when they need help. Some departments have very limited outpatient care. For example, outpatient visits to the long-term care and rehabilitation departments are usually associated with in-patient care, i.e. in-patients receiving pre- or post-treatment as outpatients. The orthopaedic department does not accept appointments by telephone; referral from a doctor is always required.

Most outpatients do not have to be hospitalised. But the outpatient/in-patient ratio varies considerably from one department to the next. According to Table 5.6, the department of infectious medicine has the lowest ratio of outpatient visits per admission (0.5).[5] It should be noted, however, that most in-patients are admitted via the outpatient clinics after having been referred there by outside doctors.

There is a waiting list for admission to most in-patient departments. The doctors' opinion as to how quickly a patient should be admitted to the hospital is expressed in terms of degree of priority. Priority classifications vary for different departments, and reflect the fact that the length of in-patient waiting lists constitutes a more serious problem in some departments than others.

TABLE 5.6

Relation between the number of outpatients and the number of admissions

	No. of patients		Ratio
	Outpatient care (a)	In-patient care (b)	(a) : (b) = (c)
Medicine	3,926	2,385	1.6
Surgery	10,892	2,805	3.9
Obstetrics and gynaecology	5,686	2,072	2.7
Paediatrics	3,084	1,813	1.7
Ear, nose and throat	6,358	1,284	5.0
Ophthalmology	6,323	372	17.0
Infectious medicine	732	1,619	0.5
Orthopaedics	2,340	548	4.3
Long-term care	425	309	1.4
Psychiatry	799	275	2.9
Child psychiatry	28	—	—
Rehabilitation	220	180	1.2

In the department of medicine, which is one of the largest at the hospital, the decision whether to admit a patient is made centrally. The assistant department chief classifies patients into four groups: extra priority, priority, regular, and light care. The latter group includes patients who are to undergo diagnostic tests. They are admitted to a special unit and are all persons who 'can take care of themselves'. Patients on the waiting list are admitted for in-patient care as follows: first, those with extra priority, then, those in the priority class; when no one in these two groups is on the waiting list, regular patients are admitted. In extreme cases, some patients without priority have had to wait as long as a year. But this applies only to patients who were offered a bed but, for one reason or another, could not accept it at that time. The usual waiting time for regular patients is around three months.

Patients on the waiting list are classified differently in other departments. Surgical patients are ranked as follows: with priority, with some priority, and regular. A similar threefold classification is used in the gynaecology, paediatric, long-term care, and rehabilitation departments. The remaining departments classify their patients in two groups: priority and regular.

The number of emergency cases admitted to the hospital can be measured on the basis of admission statistics for Saturdays, Sundays, and holidays (when most admissions are emergencies). As an approximation, we can assume that the number of emergency cases admitted is as large as the number admitted on adjacent weekdays. This method was used in setting up Table 5.7. But the total number of emergencies is much greater because many can be treated as outpatients. We were only able to obtain statistics for two departments. About 40 per cent of the emergencies to the department of medicine were hospitalised. The corresponding figure in the ophthalmology department was 3.1 per cent.

Thus, there is a clear relationship between the size of waiting lists and the number of emergencies admitted. The long waiting list in the department of medicine, for example, means that some patients have to wait such a long time that they are finally admitted as emergencies. This also implies that doctors in outpatient clinics have to treat cases that should be admitted for in-patient care.

Variations in work load

The hospital's workload varies a great deal. Since many of the variations are eliminated because of waiting lists, it is difficult to measure variations

144

TABLE 5.7

Emergencies in different departments, with variations and proportion of emergencies admitted for in-patient care (1965).

Clinic	Average no. of patients admitted per Saturday, Sunday, and holiday	Standard deviation	Relative standard deviation $\sigma\ x{:}x.\ 100$	Average no. of patients admitted per weekday	No. admitted per weekend or holiday in % of the no. admitted per weekday
Medicine	4.03	1.91	47.4	7.62	52.9
Surgery	3.51	1.87	53.3	9.49	37.0
Obstetrics and gynaecology					
Gynaecology	2.03	1.65	81.4	7.25	28.0
Obstetrics	3.82	2.12	55.5	6.46	59.1
Paediatrics	3.24	1.98	61.1	5.71	56.7
Ear, nose and throat	1.64	1.75	106.7	4.33	37.9
Ophthalmology	0.27	0.54	200.0	1.34	20.1
Infectious medicine	2.97	1.95	65.7	5.07	58.6
Chest	0.29	0.55	189.7	1.75	16.6
Orthopaedics	0.35	0.79	225.7	2.00	17.5
Long-term care	0.07	0.26	371.4	1.18	5.9
Psychiatry	0.27	0.70	259.3	0.96	28.1
Rehabilitation	0.20*	0.85	425.0	0.62	32.3
Total	22.69	6.28	27.7	53.78	42.2

*) This figure is misleading because patients are often admitted over the weekend for tests to be performed on Monday.

145

on the basis of production statistics. The three most important variations are epidemics, seasonal variations, and variations in emergency treatment.

Epidemics arise more or less randomly, though some show a certain amount of periodicity, e.g. scarlet fever and pneumonia. The most important variations are shown in Fig. 5.5, which traces the daily census in the department of infectious medicine during a seven-year period. The curve is probably evened out to some extent due to a more restrictive admissions policy as the department approaches full capacity, or when there is a staff shortage.

Seasonal variations can be seen in the department of surgery's statistics on the number of first visits to outpatient units (Fig. 5.6). Prior to May 1965, the department had no appointment system for first visits so that the number of patients examined depended on the number appearing on any given day. There were probably more patients than are shown here because, when the load was extremely heavy, patients were either sent away or got tired of waiting and left. Comparisons between 1964 and 1965 show that seasonal variations are also rather similar, with heavy decreases during the summer and immediately before the Christmas holidays. Patients simply 'don't have time to be sick on these two occasions'. Other departments show different seasonal cycles.

The emergency load, i.e. on units within the hospital designated to take care of 'acutely ill' patients, also varies considerably (see Table 5.7). We studied this by measuring the number of patients admitted to different in-patient units in the hospital on weekends and public holidays; acutely ill patients are usually the only ones admitted on these days. According to this method of measurement, the departments with the largest emergency loads are medicine, surgery, gynaecology and obstetrics, paediatrics and infectious medicine, all of which have an average of more than two emergency admissions per 24 hours.

Of the 'acute departments', gynaecology registers the most uneven patient flows, followed by infectious medicine, paediatrics, obstetrics, and the surgical and medical departments. To some extent, the ear, nose and throat department can also be regarded as an 'acute department', and exhibits large variations. It is difficult to measure variations in the other departments since the number of 'acutely ill' patients admitted is so small (see Table 5.7, column 3).

We can also measure the extent to which a department can be regarded as an acute department by relating the average number of patients admitted per weekend and holiday to the average number admitted on weekdays. The closer that these figures approximate (in this instance, the closer they are to 100 per cent), the greater is the proportion of the patient flow

146

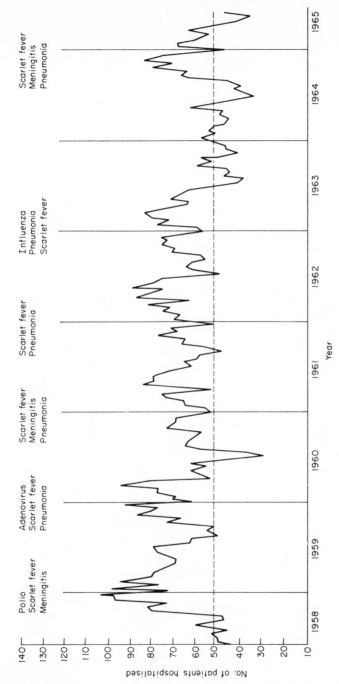

Fig. 5.5   No. of beds occupied in the department of infectious medicine on the first and fifteenth of every month 1958-1965.[6]

147

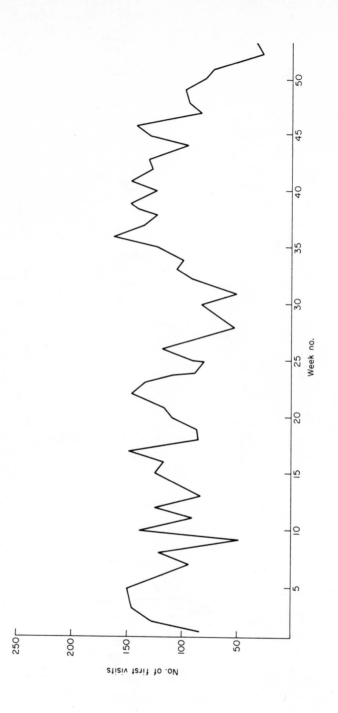

Fig. 5.6   No. of first visits to the surgical outpatient clinic.[7]

148

requiring immediate treatment. Measured in this way, the medical, obstetrics, paediatrics, and infectious medicine departments receive the largest number of patients requiring immediate treatment (see Table 5.7).

The hospital's technology

Types of components

The hospital contains different kinds of components: medical care, administrative, and others. Medical care can be divided into a wide variety of productive subcomponents, which have to be indentified and classified in order to describe the hospital's technology.

The list of the personnel categories at General Hospital provides a good picture of the variety to be found in the components. There are about fifty categories covering four groups: medical and nursing, administrative, maintenance and other personnel (see Table 5.8). But, for the reasons given below, we decided not to use these job categories in our classification.

When describing the working components, it is often desirable to deal with pairs, or groups, which work closely together, such as surgical teams, nursing teams in an outpatient unit, personnel on a ward unit, etc. It is also easier to describe the work performed by teams or groups than to give an account of what an individual does.

An employee often performs a number of quite different tasks and can be regarded as part of several components. A typical example is the department chief who sometimes works in the outpatient clinic, sometimes as adviser to junior doctors in relation to in-patient care, sometimes as part of a surgical team, etc. The hospital is divided into seventeen departmental components (including service), each headed by a department chief (see Fig. 3.2). But this classification is also insufficient for our purposes.

We discovered that people at the hospital had fairly definite ideas as to what should be regarded as distinct types of components. Table 5.9 resulted when the hospital director and some department chiefs were asked to indicate the types of 'productive units within the hospital classified in as much detail as possible, so that each type contains units which perform the same types of tasks'.

Our interviewees divided the hospital into clinical departments and central service components. These, in turn, were divided into the following subcomponents: outpatient treatment units, in-patient nursing units, and internal service units. On this basis, General Hospital contains four-

149

teen clinical departments and thirty central service components. The fourteen clinical departments have fourteen outpatient treatment units, forty-four in-patient nursing units, and thirty-four internal service components (see Table 5.10).

TABLE 5.8

Categories in General Hospital's personnel budget

Medical staff	Administrative staff
Department chief.	Hospital director
Senior dentist	Assistant to the director
Deputy department chief	Accountant
Assistant senior dentist	Assistant
Chief junior doctor	Secretary
Junior doctor	Personnel manager
Nurse (charge nurse, laboratory	Personnel assistant
nurse, X-ray nurse, assisting nurse,	
etc.)	*Maintenance staff*
Midwife	Chief engineer
Physiotherapist	Furnace man
Occupational therapist	Porter
Medical secretary	Carpenter
X-ray assistant	Painter
Laboratory assistant	Electrician
Assistant nurse	Repairman
Student nurse	Gardener
Nursing auxiliary	Kitchen supervisor
Bather	Kitchen personnel
Pharmacist	Bakery personnel
Nursery school teacher	Switchboard operator
Audiology assistant	Maid
Psychologist	Waitress
Tutor	Messenger
Medical technician	
Assistant medical technician	
Precision-tool mechanic	*Other personnel*
Photographer	Chief nurse
Cast technician	Nursing supervisor
Engineer	Social worker

150

TABLE 5.9

Main working components at General Hospital

Main components		Subcomponents			
		Outpatient treatment units	In-patient nursing units	Internal service units	Other
Clinical department	14	14	44	34	
Central service components	30	5	1		37.5
	44	19	45	34	37.5

The thirty central service components can, to some extent, be subdivided in the same way. This yields five central outpatient treatment units and a central in-patient unit (intensive care and postoperative care). There are also 37.5 other central service components which are not distributed among specific departments (see Table 5.11).

The clinical departments' various service components are shown in Table 5.12.

Degree of self-regulation

The hospital has a great many technical aids. Degree of self-regulation is an important property of these aids, and determines some of the demands made on the hospital administration. Those of the hospital's activities in which production is relatively standardised are undergoing increasing mechanisation, and even automation. Some production phases having been completely transferred to machines. This is true of medical activities in the X-ray department, central laboratory, and intensive care unit. We tried to classify the technical aids recently acquired into three categories (Table 5.13). Two of the investments in category 1, and nine in category 2 refer to the central laboratory. Nine investments in category 2 were designated for the X-ray department, and three for the intensive care unit.

Table 5.13 shows, clearly, that with but a few exceptions, medical care is still a handicraft. The most recent equipment acquired by the departments is almost exclusively made up of various kinds of tools, i.e. technical aids which require control by a human hand. The most important

TABLE 5.10

Clinical departments and their subcomponents at General Hospital

Main components	Subcomponents		
Clinical departments	Outpatient clinics	In-patient nursing units	Service components within the main component
Medicine	1	4	Clinical chemical laboratory, treatment unit (ECG)
Surgery	1	4	Operating rooms
Ear, nose and throat	1	1	Operating rooms, audiology laboratory
Ophthalmology	1	1	Operating rooms
Obstetrics and gynaecology	1	3.5	Operating rooms, prenatal clinic, delivery
Paediatrics	1	2	Child health centre, cerebral palsy unit
Infectious medicine	1	7	
Psychiatry	1	5	Clinical chemical laboratory, treatment unit (ECG), psychologist, social worker, occupational therapist
Chest	1 (allergy)	2	X-ray unit, clinical chemical laboratory, allergy laboratory, occupational therapist, physiotherapist, chest X-ray unit
Rehabilitation	1	1	Social worker, occupational therapist, physiotherapist, training kitchen
Long-term care	1	10	Social worker, occupational therapist, physiotherapist
Orthopaedics	1	2	Operating rooms, orthopaedic workshop, social worker
Child psychiatry	1	1	Psychologist, social worker
X-ray and radiotherapy	1	0.5	Department chief for therapy and diagnosis combined
Total	14	44	34

152

TABLE 5.11

Central service components and their subcomponents at General Hospital

| Main components | Subcomponents | | |
	Outpatient	In-patient nursing units	Other units
X-ray diagnosis	1		Department chief for therapy and diagnosis combined
Dental clinic	1		
Central laboratory	1		Department chief for central laboratory and blood bank combined
Blood bank	1		
Anaesthetics and intensive care		1	
Outpatient surgical unit			1
Medical supplies			1
Oxygen supply			1
Bath unit			1
Photo department			1
Central sterilisation department			1 1
Autopsy and morgue			1
Occupational therapy			4 (For departments which do not have their own staff)
Social worker			3 (idem)
Physiotherapist			9.5 (idem)
Night reception	1		
Machine room			1
Paint workshop			1
Carpentry workshop			1
Furnace room			1
Porters			1
Grounds maintenance			1
Central kitchen			1
Switchboard			1
Housekeeping department			1
Central storeroom			1
Central cloakroom			1
Library			1
Administration			1
Total	5	1	37.5

TABLE 5.12

Internal service components of clinical departments at General Hospital

Components	Number
Surgical units	5
Social workers	5
Occupational therapists	4
Physiotherapists	3
Clinical chemistry laboratories (small)	3
Treatment units	2
Psychologists	2
Prenatal care, delivery units, paediatric centre, CP-unit, chest X-ray unit, allergy laboratory, X-ray department, training kitchen, orthopaedic workshop, audiology laboratory	10
Total	34

TABLE 5.13

Classification of 107 recently acquired technical aids for medical activities[8]

Type of aids for information processing, surveillance, examination, or treatment of patients or tests	Number	%	Value (thousands of cr.)	%
1 Self-regulating aids with the ability to adapt their functioning after or during the processing of results obtained	3	2.8	114	7.4
2 Preadjustable aids set by hand, after which they carry out one or several simultaneous or successive processes	25	23.4	678	43.8
3 Aids controlled by hand which carry out one or several simultaneous or successive processes	79	73.8	755	48.8
	107		1,547	

154

exception is the medical unit's cardioverter.[9] But, even in this case, a doctor has to supervise treatment.

Predictability

Predictability of the production processes denotes the ability of those in control to make reliable predictions of the course of these processes. This factor is interesting from several points of view. In medicine, there is often a significant difference between being able to predict the amount of time which one or more measures require, and the time actually required to attain a given result. There is probably also a large difference between being able to predict the result obtained, and predicting the measures taken to achieve it. Our initial studies included many examples of differences in doctors' ability to make predictions. For example, a doctor can be fairly certain of the final outcome of treatment, but uncertain of the amount of time required. In other cases, a doctor can be fairly certain of discharging a patient within a certain time, but uncertain as to the outcome of treatment.

We measured the predictability of production processes at General Hospital in two ways. First, we studied predictability with respect to the time for which a patient would remain hospitalised. Second, we investigated predictability in relation to the length of a surgical operation. Because most doctors at General Hospital treat several patients simultaneously in outpatient clinics, we could not measure predictability of the length of treatment times there; these doctors also have to cope with many disturbances (telephone calls, in-patients, consultation with colleagues, etc.). This implies that the actual treatment time cannot be compared with the expected length of treatment time in evaluating the predictability of production processes. Another factor is that the length of treatment time in outpatient clinics is to a large extent influenced by the doctor himself.

Studies of the predictability of the time for which a patient would be hospitalised were complicated by an increase in the doctor's ability to make predictions during the course of a patient's treatment. Figure 5.7 shows a junior doctor's daily forecast of the length of a patient's stay from the time he was admitted until he was discharged ten days later. But this example is not wholly representative. The total amount of the time involved depends on many factors that the doctor is in no position to evaluate. For example, the total length of time might be related to having tests performed in the laboratory, making X-ray examinations according to plan, obtaining a bed for the patient in a convalescent home, etc.

155

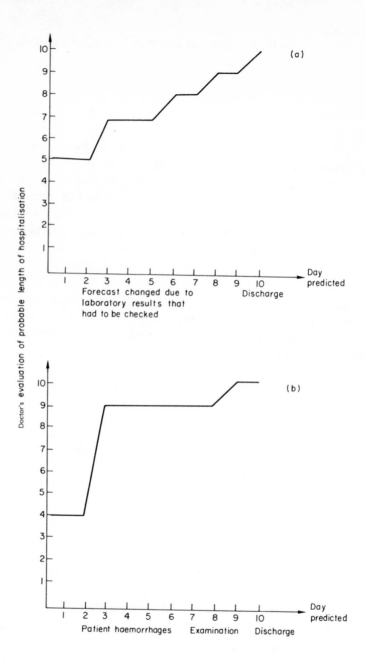

Fig. 5.7   Evaluation of probable length of hospitalisation for patients in the department of medicine at General Hospital.

156

Another type of difficulty relates to predicting the effect of treatment. This kind of forecast is also vague at first. Doctors thought it almost meaningless to answer the question: 'What do you think is the probable length of time that this patient will remain in the hospital?' Their estimates were full of reservations. But, as treatment progressed, forecasts as to the time for which a patient would have to stay in hospital became more reliable.

We avoided the difficulty inherent in successive improvement in forecasts by asking some doctors (in medicine, surgery, and paediatrics) to predict how long all the patients in their units on a given day would have to remain in hospital (see Fig. 5.8). The results yielded very low predictability. Unfortunately, we could not get the doctors to participate in a more extensive study which would have provided statistical evidence of the differences between various departments and of the discharge predictability with regard to different groups of patients.

In studying the predictability of the length of surgical and orthopaedic operations; we found that we could greatly increase the surgeons forecasting ability by providing him with statistics on earlier similar cases, and information on the outcome of previous forecasts. Figure 5.9 indicates that forecasting ability varies considerably from one case to the next. The length of some operations such as appendectomies or variocotomies can

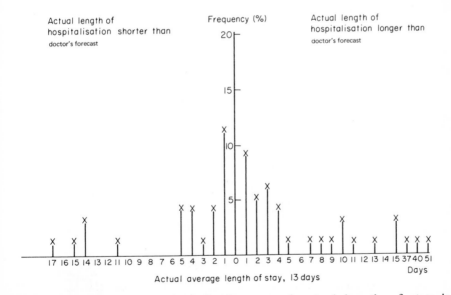

Fig. 5.8 Deviation from doctor's forecast of actual length of stay in the hospital.

157

be predicted fairly accurately. But the length of other operations can vary a great deal. There is a high degree of uncertainty as to the length of time which a surgeon predicts as necessary for a stomach operation.

It seems surprising that the physician's ability to make predictions increases as treatment progresses, especially as we restricted our study to experienced surgeons. It is difficult to interpret the results reported in Fig. 5.9; they indicate the forecasting success of physicians who received limited training in predicting the length of an operation. We might ask whether predictions with respect to the length of hospitalisation could also be improved by training the physicians in this matter.

Service content

Service means production that takes place only in conjunction with customer (patient) contact. The service content of the production process can be measured in many different ways, e.g. working time, cost, etc.

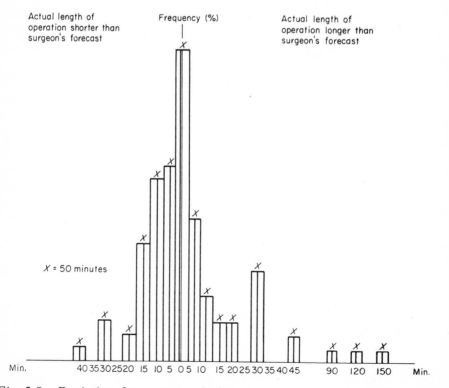

Fig. 5.9   Deviation from surgeon's forecast of actual length of operation.

158

Precise measurements of service content require extensive time and motion studies which could not be performed for our study. We thought that a relatively reliable and simple method of measurement could be based on determining the proportion of employees having regular contacts with patients (see Table 5.14).

Some 80 per cent of the employees at the hospital were found to have regular contacts with patients. This seems to be a high figure when compared to industrial firms. Measured in this way, departments with in-patient units exhibit a service content of between 90 and 100 per cent.

The production system

Size of the production system

The size of the production system refers simply to the number of components. Measurements of the size of the production system have to be based on a given level of analysis. If we study the most basic level, we find that each employee is a component. But, as mentioned in connection with our classification of components, most people working in the hospital have definite ideas about its components (our experience from other production systems is similar). Thus, according to this classification, the hospital's production system was composed of 114 subcomponents at the beginning, and 135.5 subcomponents at the end of our study (see Table 5.9). This indicates a rapid increase in the size of the hospital during the period in which our study was in progress. We can get an even better idea of this growth by looking at conditions ten and twenty years ago (Table 5.15). The production system is nearly four times larger than it was twenty years ago and has grown by 25 per cent during the past ten years. The number of outpatient treatment units has increased with the establishment of new specialties. Internal service components have also expanded in all units.

Specialisation and diversity

The 'assortment' of services which the hospital is supposed to provide, and the large variations in demands on the hospital, prompted us to investigate the degree of diversity in its components. A wide assortment and variations in demand are easy to handle in an organisation where everyone can

159

do everything. Production capacity can be adapted, for instance, by varying the number of staff in relation to demand. The greater the degree of specialisation among components, the more that other means such as extended planning and closer control have to be used to attain the flexibility required.

Our interest in the diversity and interchangeability of components also increased during our initial contacts with the hospital. We saw examples of

TABLE 5.14

Service content of the production units for the components at General Hospital[10]

Clinical department or equivalent	No. of employees	Employees with daily patient contact	Ratio of (3) : (2) as %
(1)	(2)	(3)	(4)
Medicine	86	80	93
Surgery	99	97	98
Obstetrics and gynaecology	82	82	100
Paediatrics	44	40	91
Ear, nose and throat	28	27	96
Ophthalmology	18	18	100
Chest	37	35	94
Long-term care	150	143	95
Psychiatry	60	54	90
Rehabilitation	12	12	100
Infectious medicine	67	62	92
Orthopaedics	29	28	96
Child psychiatry	21	21	100
Anaesthetics	23	23	100
X-ray	47	37	79
Central laboratory	42	21	50
All medical and nursing staff	845	780	92
Administration	19	0	0
Maintenance staff	108	0	0
Other staff	55	42	76
Entire hospital	1,027	822	80

160

TABLE 5.15

Three measurements showing the growth of the production system

		1945	1955	1965
1 No. of components with a department chief as supervisor	Total	7	10	17
2 Clinical departments		6	7	14
Central service components		15	23	30
	Total	21	30	44
3 Outpatient treatment units (including nights)		9	12	19
In-patient nursing units		10.5	15.5	45
Service components within departments		6	9	34
Other		12	17	37.5
	Total	37.5	53.5	135.5

the way in which doctors took care of emergencies that appeared to be far outside their normal area of competence. Moreover, the charge nurse stressed the importance of being able to deploy nurses in fairly radical ways in the event of illness, or absence for other reasons. We also understood that there were definite limits on the degree of interchangeability. An experienced nurse could never be considered a substitute for a junior doctor and administrative staff were seldom transferred to nursing units.

We tried to obtain a more detailed picture of these conditions by undertaking more interviews and more systematic measurements. But the problem was complex, particularly because of the large number of component types and the relatively large differences between them. Conditions were typified primarily by very strong professional stratification. Members of one professional group cannot, and are unwilling to, perform tasks, which they feel belong to another group. This situation is mainly due to educational differences and the hospital's social structure.

Social strata can be observed, for example, in the hospital's dining arrangements, doctors eat in a separate room from the rest of the staff. In the main dining-room, office staff, student nurses, and other employees all eat in their own 'corners', while nurses, nursing auxiliaries, physiotherapists and social workers form groups, in another part.

Since the limitations on interchangeability are the result of educational and social conditions, and not mechanisation they are less clear, and more flexible, than those in an industrial firm, and are often disregarded in

161

emergencies. Many employees complained about 'increasing specialisation'. They said that the functions of each component used to be broader (though knowledge of specific details was less profound), and that this was highly advantageous. But they also stressed that General Hospital's high degree of specialisation provided distinctive competence as compared, for example, with a smaller hospital.

Despite professional stratification, rigidly limiting mobility between different professional groups, there is significant interchangeability within each group, and almost complete interchangeability in some groups (see Table 5.16). In the daily routine of an in-patient unit, there is a distinct division of work, though conscious efforts are made to give everyone the same amount of experience. This is achieved by rotation and division of the tasks involving little specialisation, the kind of work performed in the various in-patient units being very similar.

Social workers are an example of a professional group with specialised education but relatively little specialisation within the group itself. Table 5.17 shows the head social worker's evaluation of her colleagues' ability, after a short training period, to give a doctor the kind of help he really wants. When we substituted a lower requirement—'to keep things running smoothly' — complete interchangeability was reported.

TABLE 5.16

A nursing supervisor's evaluation of the ability of 15 randomly chosen nursing auxiliaries to perform another job for a limited period of time after one week's training.

Can replace	A	B	C	D	E	F	G	H	I	J	K	L	M	N	O	Remarks
A		X	X	X			X	X	X	X	X	X	X	X	X	
B							X									
C	X	X		X			X	X	X	X	X	X	X	X	X	
D	X	X	X				X	X	X	X	X	X	X	X	X	
E					X											
F	X	X	X	X	X		X	X	X	X	X	X	X	X	X	
G		X														Incapable
H	X	X	X	X			X		X	X	X	X	X	X	X	
I	X	X	X	X			X	X		X	X		X	X	X	Physically
J	X	X	X	X			X	X	X		X	X	X	X		
K											X					Psychologically
L	X	X	X	X			X	X	X	X	X		X	X	X	
M	X	X	X	X		X	X	X	X	X	X	X		X	X	
N	X	X	X	X			X	X	X	X	X	X	X		X	
O	X	X	X	X			X	X	X	X	X	X	X	X		

162

TABLE 5.17

Head social worker's evaluation of her colleagues' ability to 'provide the help a doctor wants' after a short training period.

Can replace/social worker	A	B	C	D	E	F
A		x	x	x	x	x
B			x			x
C		x				x
D		x	x		?	x
E		x	x	x	x		x
F		x	x			

X = denotes interchangeability
? = denotes uncertainty

The chief nurse, who evaluated 25 randomly chosen nurses (Table 5.18), was very doubtful as to the ability of some nurses to 'change jobs'. This is also supported by the specialised education and training of the following nursing groups: midwives, laboratory, X-ray, surgical and medical duty nurses. Table 5.18 also shows that the interchangeability of certain subgroups is more limited than others.

As expected, the greatest degree of specialisation occurs among doctors. This specialisation is quite clear-cut and implies that certain types of operations, diagnoses, or therapy can be performed exclusively by specific individuals. But this is only half the truth. As well as specialising, all doctors are experienced and knowledgeable in many areas where their background is more or less the same. Many of them also have profound knowledge of some 'subspecialty'.[11]

Interchangeability within a group could be measured in terms of the quotient of the number of possible changes divided by the maximum number of changes if everyone in a specific professional group could replace one another. The results are shown in Table 5.19. Measurements of this kind, however, do not prove that personnel could be interchanged to the extent indicated in this part of our study. What we actually measured was some kind of technical interchangeability. The chief nurse said: 'In my opinion, the nurses/nursing auxiliaries do not believe that they are this interchangeable, nor do they want to move about from one job to the next'.

The staff themselves have a more modest estimate of their interchange-

163

ability, and usually do not want to change jobs. In addition, the situation on the labour market today gives them an opportunity to achieve their demands. Later we shall describe the way in which changes in participant conditions—such as staff demands for more leisure time and less on-call service—require increased interchangeability. The demand for interchangeability is a growing problem at the hospital. Many employees also feel that interchangeability of jobs is becoming progressively less frequent and blame specialisation for this trend. The personnel department, chief nurse, and nursing supervisors devote a great deal of their time to convincing, persuading or finding personnel (in Industry Town) who are willing to

TABLE 5.18

Chief nurse's evaluation of the technical ability of 25 randomly chosen nurses to perform another job satisfactorily for a limited period of time after a week's training.

Can replace Nurse		A	B	C	D	E	F	G	H	I	J	K	L	M	N	O	P	Q	R	S	T	U	V	X	Y	Z
Out-	A		X	X					X		X															
patient	B	X		X					X	X	X		X	X	X	X			X	X	X					X
treat-	C	X	X		?	?	?	?	X	X	X	X			X	X	X	X	X	X		X				X
ment	D	X	X			X			X		X													X	X	X
unit	E	X	X		X				X		X			X		X			X	X	X			X	X	X
	F	X	X	X				X	X	X	X	X	X	X	X	X	X	X	X	X	X	X				X
	G	X	X	X			X		X	?	X	?	?	?	?	?	?	?	?	?	?					X
	H	X	X	X		?				X	X		X	X	X	X	X	X	X	X	X			X	X	X
	I	X	X	X					X		X	X	X	X	X	X	X	X	X	X	X	X				X
	J	X	X	X	X	X			X	X					X	X								X	X	X
In-	K			X					X		X		X	X						X	X					X
patient	L	X	X						X		X		X	X	X				X							X
nursing	M	X	X	X					X		X		X		X	X		X	X	X	X					X
unit	N	X	X						X		X		X	X		X		X			X					X
	O	X	X	X	?	?	?	?	?	X	X	X	X	X	X	X		X	X	X	X	X				X
	P	X	X	X					X	X	X	X		X	X	X		X	X	X	X					X
	Q	X	X	X					X	X	X	X	X	X	X	X	X		X	X	X	X				X
	R	X	X						X	X	X		X	X	X	X		X								X
	S	X	X	X					X	X	X	X	X	X		X	X	X	X		X					X
	T	X	X	X	?	?	?	?	?	X	X	X	X	X	X	X	X	X	X	X	X			X	X	X
Special	U	X	X						X																	
unit	V			X					X	X	X															
	X	X	X	X	X	X	X	X	X	X	X													X	X	
	Y	X	X			X	X	X	X	X		X	X	X	X	X		X	X	X	X					X
	Z	X	X	X	X	X	X	X	X	X	X	X	X	X	X		X	X	X	X				X	X	

? denotes uncertainty
X denotes interchangeability

164

TABLE 5.19

Interchangeability index for different personnel categories.

Personnel category	Total no. of possible changes (a)	Real no. of possible changes (b)	Interchangeability index (b) : (a) (c)
Nursing auxiliaries	210	142	0.67
Social workers	30	20	0.67
Nurses	600	311	0.52
on in-patient nursing units	90	69	0.77
in special services	20	5	0.25
in outpatient units	90	54	0.60

help out in units with staff shortages. Monetary inducements which could make flexible jobs more attractive are also lacking.[12]

Degree of autonomy of the hospital and its subsystems

We measured the degree of autonomy of the various subsystems on the basis of the classification used at the hospital, i.e. in terms of the division into clinical departments. We tried to measure autonomy by calculating the quotient of the cost of services supplied from outside the departments, divided by the salary costs of each unit. A similar calculation was made for the hospital as a whole. Table 5.20 shows that, as a whole, the hospital is a highly autonomous system. The medical and surgical departments have the lowest degrees of autonomy, since patients pass through them on their way to other special units in the hospital. The psychiatry and ophthalmology departments do not depend on central services (such as the central laboratory) as much as other departments do—thus, their relatively higher degree of autonomy.

Capacity

We tried to indentify bottlenecks and assess waiting lists on the basis of a questionnaire to the department chiefs. We also interviewed nurses and junior doctors, again to identify bottlenecks, particularly the capacity of department chiefs and deputy department chiefs. The results of the first-mentioned study are shown in Table 5.21. The waiting time for an out-patient appointment is longest in the department of psychiatry. This is due to the scarcity of psychiatrists and to the considerable amount of time which doctors in this field need for outpatient care. In contrast, in the surgical department many cases can be treated per unit of time.

Since many of the surgical cases admitted are often highly complicated, there tends to be a long list of patients waiting for operations which are not of an acute nature. Another problem in this context is the difficulty or impossibility of discharging cases to convalescent or nursing homes,etc. There is a priority ranking for in-patients so that cancer cases, for example, receive priority (two to three days' waiting time) while gall bladder cases have to wait longer. This problem is fairly serious in the department of medicine, where 27 per cent of beds are occupied by such cases.

The orthopaedic department exhibits another pattern. The amount of outpatient care is adapted to the capacity of surgical and in-patient units.

TABLE 5.20

Coefficient of dependency for in-patient and outpatient units — quotient of costs for services supplied from outside the department and salaries in the department.[13]

Clinical departments	Coefficient of dependency
Medicine	0.70
Surgery	0.83
Obstetrics and gynaecology	0.47
Paediatrics	0.41
Ear, nose and throat	0.49
Ophthalmology	0.21
Infectious diseases	0.34
Orthopaedic	0.83
Long-term care	0.31
Psychiatry	0.21
Rehabilitation	0.64
Entire hospital	0.07

TABLE 5.21

Waiting times for in-patient and outpatient care

Clinical department	In-patient care		Outpatient care	
	Waiting time (days)	No. of persons waiting	Average no. of patients treated per day	Of whom do not require hospitalisation
Medicine	10-30	162	96	24
Surgery	3-4	450	95	30
Long-term care	7	287	161	26
Chest	5-10	41	40	9
Psychiatry	300	10	24	0
Orthopaedics	75	33	20	0
Others	98	180	206	10
Total	498-524	1.163	642	99

This can be done mainly because orthopaedic conditions are seldom fatal. But it also means long outpatient lists, though the number of people waiting for in-patient care is usually both manageable and foreseeable. Some orthopaedic patients are also treated in the surgical outpatient department.

In sum, the most characteristic feature of the hospital's capacity is the great difference between departments. Waiting time for the surgical outpatient clinic is three to four days, but 450 persons are on the waiting list for in-patient care. Waiting time for the psychiatry clinic is 300 days for outpatients, but the waiting list for in-patient care contains only 10 names. Waiting time for outpatients in the medical clinic is not long, but 162 persons were waiting to be admitted and 27 patients could have been discharged if post-hospital care could have been arranged.

Department chiefs, junior doctors, and a number of nurses were asked the following two questions: 'What parts of the department are so overloaded that treatment of in-patients is sometimes delayed?' and 'What services from other departments, service units, or agencies outside the hospital involve waiting times that delay treatment of in-patients?' The results support our general impression from a number of interviews and observations, i.e. that (with only a few exceptions) there is sufficient capacity in service units so that in-patient care is not delayed. The outpatient service units are generally overloaded. This is one explanation for the long outpatient waiting lists in all clinics. The 60 people asked about reasons for delays said that 45 per cent could be attributed to X-ray

167

TABLE 5.22

Do the doctors constitute bottlenecks?

Question to doctors (deputy department chiefs and junior doctors):
How often are you so busy that treatment of in-patients is delayed?

	No. of respondents	%
Daily	3	8.3
Every week	7	19.4
Monthly	7	19.4
Twice a year	—	—
Every other year	1	2.8
Never or almost never	9	25.0
Never	8	22.2
No answer	1	2.8
	36	99.9

Question to charge nurses:
How often are the doctors so busy that treatment of in-patients is delayed?

	No. of respondents	%
Daily	4	9.5
Every week	9	21.4
Monthly	2	4.8
Twice a year	—	—
Every other year	—	—
Never or almost never	17	40.5
No answer	10	23.8
	42	100.0

Question to doctors (department chiefs, deputy department chiefs, and junior doctors):
How often are the department chiefs and deputy department chiefs in your department so busy that treatment of in-patients is delayed?

	No. of respondents	%
Daily	4	7.5
Every week	5	9.4
Monthly	4	7.5
Twice a year	3	5.7
Every other year	1	1.9
Never or almost never	12	22.6
Never	18	34.0
No answer	6	11.3
	53	99.9

168

diagnosis, 20 per cent to a lack of long-term care facilities and 15 per cent to psychiatric consultation. As for conditions within the departments, 30 per cent mentioned 'shortage of staff', and 15 per cent said that insufficient capacity in surgery tended to cause delays.[14]

Our initial interviews gave us the impression that the doctors' heavy workloads and intensive involvement in outpatient care sometimes led to delays in treatment of in-patients, lack of time for planning examinations and treatment, delays in discharging patients, etc. Questions to the doctors and nurses involved are not a reliable method of studying these conditions, but owing to a lack of resources for more detailed investigations, we asked the doctors: 'How often are you so busy that treatment of in-patients is delayed?' and the nurses: 'How often are the doctors so busy that treatment of in-patients is delayed?' Some 47 per cent of the doctors questioned thought that their work in the in-patient units is never, or almost never, delayed because they are too busy (see Table 5.22). The doctors were also asked how often department chiefs and deputy department chiefs were so busy that treatment of in-patients was delayed. Some 57 per cent said that this never, or almost never, occurred.

Notes

[1] The height of the column is proportional to the number of patients cared for, the width to the average cost, and the area to the total cost of care provided.

[2] This refers to concrete subsystems as opposed to the abstract systems discussed at the beginning of chapter 2. See J. G. Miller, Living Systems: Basic Concepts, *Behavioral Science* 10.3, 1965, pp. 193-237.

[3] The patient's possibilities of being treated by the doctor of his choice are extremely limited since private outpatient care was abolished at the hospital (see note 7 to chapter 4).

[4] Different departments have introduced light care. There is, for instance, a medical diagnostic observation unit, a puerperal unit in the obstetric department, and a light-care unit in the orthopaedic and rehabilitation departments.

[5] Owing to poor facilities in the department of infectious medicine, the department chief also has a private practice in town. This probably affects the number of outpatient visits.

[6] Average no. of beds occupied 59; standard deviation 12; range 75.

[7] Average no. of patients hospitalised 105.6; standard deviation 31.3; range 136. Data refer to 1964.

[8] This classification was made by a department chief who was specially selected because of his good perspective of all departments. He classified all recently acquired technical aids except a few designated for X-ray and the central laboratory (which were classified by department chiefs in each of these units). Another department chief classified them in the same way which indicated that the first classification had good reliability.

[9] Technical aids introduced into the hospital are usually motivated by the fact that diagnosis and therapy can be carried out that would otherwise not be possible without this equipment, i.e. there is an improvement in quality. Sometimes, but not always, the new equipment facilitates or speeds up certain tasks.

[10] These figures are estimates based on a study of personnel records.

[11] Interchangeability with respect to doctors is closely related to the interchangeability of clinical departments. The latter could be measured from answers to the following question: 'On any given day, ask the department chief to evaluate the possibilities of transferring treatment of all hospitalised patients to another department without medical disadvantages.'

[12] Sociological studies indicate that the degree of impersonality in contacts between persons in an organisation can be regarded as an aid in

170

facilitating interchangeability among the personnel. People at Swedish hospitals generally do not address each other by name but use 'names' related to their jobs (i.e. titles such as doctor, nurse, 'little' nurse, social worker, etc.).

[13]   Consultation costs are not included.

[14]   This part of the study was carried out in September 1965. The child psychiatry department was not yet in operation and is therefore not included in tne results. Conditions in the child psychiatry department are more or less the same as in the adult psychiatry unit, i.e. there is a long outpatient waiting list and a relatively small number of patients waiting to be hospitalised.

6 Administration of the Hospital's Participant Groups

The relations between the hospital's participant groups were described in chapter 4. In chapter 2, we said that these relationships make demands on management which, in turn, have to be fulfilled to achieve efficiency. Some kind of participant administration, i.e. measures aimed at influencing the participants, is required to fulfil these demands. We intend to formulate these demands in more detail, and then examine how the hospital is equipped to meet them. This analysis is based on our observations after having studied the hospital's participant relations, but before we had established more than unsystematic and superficial contact with the hospital's management. We then describe the situation at the hospital itself, to try to evaluate whether the hospital's participant administration is able to meet the demands of the situation.

Before beginning our analysis, we have to distinguish between strategic planning, planning for resource procurement, and policy formulation. This differentiation is based on the following description of the way in which some of the fundamental decisions on participant administration are made in an organisation.

The management in every organisation, consciously or unconsciously, chooses a strategy, i.e. a combination of participants and institutions for resolving conflicts. Sometimes, this strategy has to be revised because of a changing environment. This can be accomplished by reviewing relations with each individual participant group, or by re-examining the strategy as a whole. The review process takes place more or less consciously. But regardless of the way in which it occurs, we call it strategic planning.

The strategy adopted is usually specified, and augmented by attitudes that are accepted as a matter of principle; these attitudes refer to the organisation's behaviour in relation to its participants. Some of the attitudes are adopted without conscious deliberation by the management of the organisation, but more often, they are formulated and prescribed—in which case they are designated the organisation's policy. Regardless of how much conscious effort goes into choosing a strategy and formulating a policy, the management often believes that it has to make quantitative estimates of the organisation's production, i.e. plan for resource procurement and contributions to be exchanged with its various participants. This plan is called a budget if it covers one or two years, or a long-term plan when it covers three to ten years.

Strategic planning

Expectations

Choosing a strategy is often said to be top management's most important task. This applies especially to an institutionalised firm which is relatively independent of its participants. But the analysis in chapter 3 indicated that the situation with regard to a hospital is quite different. A hospital does not associate with most of its participants on a market basis but is linked to them through legislation, long-term agreements, and social norms. Thus, we did not expect the hospital management to question or feel obliged to reconsider the hospital's strategy. Even if the management—as private individuals—thought that some aspects of policy were unsuitable, they would still be obliged (in their capacity as members of the county council, the board of trustees, or as department chiefs) to adhere loyally to the objectives prescribed by government commissions, Parliament, the National Board of Health and Welfare, and the Association of County Councils. Instead of strategic planning which would challenge objectives and the mix of participants involved in the hospital, we expected the hospital's management to try to anticipate the demands and future actions which would be stipulated by the participants in terms of laws, instructions, agreements, etc.

The hospital management does have some freedom of action, and the fact that strategic planning was being performed at all was a major exception to our general expectations. We did expect strategic planning to occur in the hospital's relations to its personnel. This was based on our knowledge of the difficulties of satisfying personnel demands and retaining personnel; also, the considerable freedom of action which the hospital has in relation to personnel (department chiefs apart). We expected to find strategic considerations with respect to hiring foreign personnel, with some recruitment abroad; changes in working methods aimed at facilitating recruitment of personnel, etc.

Product assortment is usually a decisive factor in terms of effective production. We expected the hospital's management to exercise its freedom of action in this area. For example, we thought that the almost unlimited product assortment would be regarded as an obstacle to

174

efficiency. Thus, we expected a regular assessment of the division of work between General Hospital and other institutions. We also anticipated policy discussions on resource allocation between in-patient and out-patient care and the status of by-products (such as education and research). The hospital management also has a certain amount of freedom of action with regard to expansion, particularly in terms of setting prior-ities for expansion into new areas of activity, and we expected this to be an important part of its strategic planning.

As for the methods applied in strategic planning, we expected matters related to staff turnover and the division of labour between General Hos-pital and other institutions to be dealt with as factual problems with unambiguous goals (such as reducing the cost of medical care, lessening the need for personnel, or increasing the 'quantity of care' produced). We thought that these kinds of issues would be handled and solved by the professional hospital management. Decisions with respect to expansion involved a conflict between the interests of different patient groups. Even if economic evaluations were possible to some extent, we expected politic-al authorities to have the greatest amount of influence on decisions involv-ing priority for politically feasible expansions.

Measurements

Strategic planning is—as we expected—not the primary task of any member of the hospital management. Some members say that the manage-ment does not usually deal with important matters at all. When we studied the matters handled by the board of trustees in 1965, the results were rather scant (see Table 6.1). Strategic matters are discussed primarily in connection with annual personnel budget negotiations. But, even in this sphere, the hospital management has limited influence.

Expansion is the most important issue in the hospital's long-term planning, and is expected to remain so during the next few years. Expan-sion not only refers to quantitative additions of new nursing units but also to selecting the specialties to be represented at General Hospital. Typical issues of this kind include the establishment and aims of the long-term care and child psychiatry units, and the addition of occupational medicine as a subspecialty in the department of medicine, introduction of X-ray therapy, health screening to be performed at the hospital, and discussions about new quarters for the bacteriology and pathology laboratories. The task of understanding the way in which strategic decisions are made was interesting, as well as difficult. Our methods consisted primarily of interviewing people working on various aspects of the planning process, and our overall interpretation is as follows. The interviews were informal and guided by a simple set of questions:

Whose initiative was it?
What opinions from different quarters influenced the decision?
Who looked for alternatives?
Who studied the consequences of different alternatives?
Who made the decision?
Who influenced the decision making?
In what respects were the organisation's objectives affected by the decisions?

According to public health laws, the County Health and Medical Services Board is required to draw up general plans for medical care. But in 1965, expansion of medical care in the county was being studied by a special committee for planning the county council's long-term investments. This study was similar to one made in 1953, when plans were drawn up for long-term expansion of General Hospital in Industry Town. The planning variables are apparent from the following questions:

What clinical departments should General Hospital in Industry Town have?
What concentration of qualified medical care should there be at General Hospital?
What concentration of costly service departments (such as the central laboratory) should there be at General Hospital?
How many beds are required in the various departments at General Hospital?

It was clear that this work was guided to a large extent by studies carried out by the central public health and medical care authorities.[1] The evaluations made did not include a determination of the extent of different health care requirements because planners have access to national forecasts. The most difficult problem seemed to involve balancing local interests for several completely equipped hospital facilities in the vicinity, and the economic and medical motives for concentrating the county's health care resources at General Hospital. A leading member of the county council put the problem this way: 'The distribution of resources between General Hospital and other units which would very much like to become small hospitals is the county council's most important task'.

176

The hospital is represented on the committee by the chairman of the board of trustees. The chairman of the committee is the head of the executive committee, and the chief of the medical staff serves as medical adviser. The person in charge of performing the study itself is an employee of the administration of the county council, not the hospital. The plan has been revised several times between 1953 (when the previous long-term plan was made) and 1965 (when the new committee was appointed). These revisions were carried out by the county council central building committee. When this committee discussed matters related to the hospital, General Hospital was represented by the chairman of the board of trustees, the hospital director, and the chief of the medical staff. Thus, the hospital's interests are supported by constant references to the 1953 plan, with demands that it be put into effect. Department chiefs also took the initiative over obtaining additional resources and bringing about other changes. These initiatives often took place through direct contacts between department chiefs and influential members of the county council. The department chiefs' association and the committee also collaborate to some extent. Our collective impression is that the board of trustees is less important than the department chiefs' group in terms of initiating strategic changes. In general, decisions made by the board of trustees are initiated by previous action or by reminders from one or several department chiefs.

Regardless of whether the county council or the department chiefs take the initiative, changes usually originate with, or have the blessings of, central public health and medical authorities (government agency, the National Board of Health and Welfare, or the Association of County Councils). General Hospital in Industry Town and the county council do not believe that they should, or could be pioneers who try out measures not yet investigated by the central authorities. However, there have been some minor deviations, as when a department structure was proposed at General Hospital which was more extensive than usual for general hospitals and in some respects corresponded to a regional hospital.

Building problems are another important aspect of long-term planning. For instance, a decision was made to give priority to plans for the department of infectious medicine because facilities there were so poor that further delays could not be tolerated.

The county council has often rejected proposals from General Hospital regarding poor facilities. Building matters predominate in the general plan for the hospital. An influential county council member said that the most important task of the general plan was to 'remain flexible'. 'If you have a multi-storey building, you have to ask yourself where the next phase is

TABLE 6.1

Matters handled during meetings of the board of trustees, 1965

Subject	Type of consideration	Reason
January		
Salary benefits in connection with introduction courses for new personnel	Report	County council's position towards previous proposals from the board
February		
Stipends for student nurses	Discussion of principles: 'What procedure should we adopt at General Hospital?'	Initiatives by other county councils required counter measures
Personnel service in the county council	Remarks based on a survey made by the Association of County Councils	Report circulated for comment from the county Health and Medical Services Board
Waiting time at outpatient clinics	Discussion	Report from HMS
Personnel administrative study	Discussion and decision to use a consultant	Initiative by the executive committee
Facilities for the department of infectious medicine	Decision to inspect building	Complaint from department chief
April		
Problems related to facilities at the hospital	Discussion and decision to make a report to the executive committee	Budget work had revealed a number of problems with respect to facilities
Family service bureau	Discussion and rejection	Report circulated for comment from HMS
Occupational medicine clinic	Discussion and approval with certain conditions	Proposal by a department chief
May		
Principles for leaves of absence	Discussion	A recent case
Male medical service personnel	Discussion	Report from HMS
ADP for store-room accounting	Report	Decision to give approval made by HMS
Punch-card registration of diagnoses and operations	Discussion and decision to establish an experimental system	Difficulties in manual processing; initiative of the chief accountant

178

Table 6.1 (continued)

June		
Centralised cleaning of the hospital	Discussion of proposal from the hospital director; appropriations requested from HMS	
Personnel budget and plans for child psychiatry department	Discussion and approval of proposal; referred to HMS	
Expanded personnel department	Discussion of study made by a consultant; proposal for personnel budget to HMS	Study proposed by the county council and hospital board
July		
X-ray examinations for personnel	Discussion of proposals for expansion	Proposal from personnel physician
September		
Daily schedule for child day-care centre	Discussion of proposal—referred to HMS	New day-care centre opened with new staff and new hours
October		
Rearrangement of in-patient units	Discussion of proposal from hospital director—referred to HMS	Increased workloads in two clinical departments
November		
Additional personnel for obstetrics and gynaecology department	Discussion of proposal by department chief—referred to HMS	Increased workload
December		
New patient cards	Request appropriation from HMS	

179

going to be located. Future expansion must not be thwarted.' The most important values influencing strategic planning involved efforts to retain all opportunities of meeting new health care needs, improving the quality of medical care, and solving staff shortage problems. Some of those we interviewed suspected that, when individual department chiefs or groups of doctors tried to get certain things accomplished, such initiatives were based on personal motives.

But it is not unusual for a department head to feel a certain responsibility for expansion in his own area of activity. What perhaps surprised us the most was that pressure from patient groups or political authorities seemed so weak. Medical check-ups were introduced through a motion in the county council—but this is an exception. Efforts to establish new specialties have sometimes been based on needs expressed by other authorities or local industries. Active campaigns from patient groups or other participants have not, to our knowledge, influenced strategic planning at General Hospital.[2]

Our expectation that the hospital's management would try to anticipate participants' demands and future actions was not met. We tried to get different people to indicate changes that they expected to occur during the next five-year period. These opinions varied a great deal.

Table 6.2 is based on interviews with some members of the hospital management and the county council and its staff. It shows that there is no consensus of opinion and that expectations are generally unclear. All members of the board of trustees were asked to respond to a questionnaire containing the same questions. One or two of them made references to earlier oral interviews, otherwise none mentioned changes other than expansion of facilities and clinics. The explanation is simple. The time allotted for work on the board (and subcommittee) was used for more urgent matters, and none was left for discussing forecasts.

We did find, however, that persons in lower supervisory positions at the hospital gave much more complete and descriptive answers to this question than did members of the board. In addition to new buildings and clinical departments, their expectations as to what would be changed at General Hospital included a more active personnel policy, technological changes (such as ADP), increased rationalisation and education, improved coordination between psychiatric and general medical care, more male employees, shorter working hours, three shifts, improved administration, etc. Of course, the board of trustees is aware of all this. The differences in answers might simply be due to the fact that the members of the board spent less time responding to the questionnaire.

The task of finding alternatives and evaluating their consequences has

180

been difficult and complex in regard to several current strategic matters. In other words, there is a considerable element of problem-solving. As in the case of initiative taking, the committee has, to a large extent, used studies and evaluations from various central agencies. The Thapper study [3] was used as the basis for a decision to reallocate tasks performed by nurses and medical service personnel. The X-ray therapy and occupational medicine units were started only after scrutiny by the National Board of Health and Welfare. In some instances, the doctors' professional organisations have

TABLE 6.2

Answers obtained during interviews with some members of the county council and hospital management about future changes

Respondent (in random order)	What changes do you think will take place during the next five years with respect to laws, rules, and recommendations now in effect at General Hospital?	What are the most important changes you think will take place at General Hospital during the next five years?
1	There won't be any changes.	New building. Division of existing specialties and establishment of new ones.
2	Reorganisation of the National Board of Health and Welfare. But I don't know anything about all this.	Larger in-patient units. Perhaps new buildings. Some centralisation from the county council
3	Decentralisation from the Board of Health and Welfare. Care of the mentally ill. Possibly also geriatrics.	Improved personnel situation. More resources for rationalisation. More highly differentiated care. Perhaps a decrease in the out-patient workload.
4	The fee structure? I haven't thought about the question.	Expansion—new specialties. Private and public clinics reduce the pressure on the hospital. Better educated medical personnel.
5	I have no opinion about this.	New specialties.
6	I don't know.	New facilities and clinics. No organisational changes.
7	I haven't thought about the question.	Expanded care of the chronically ill. New specialties. Coordination with psychiatric care. No organisational changes, except perhaps for those which occur in the county council, can affect General Hospital.
8	I don't know.	We have the specialties we need. I don't know what's lacking. Better educated personnel?

181

similar status due to their long-term ability to evaluate the speed with which competent candidates for new departmental head positions can be expected to become available.

But these kinds of central studies seldom provide a sufficient basis for executing important changes at General Hospital. Execution of the Thapper study's proposal to allocate tasks performed by nurses, assistant nurses and nursing auxiliaries, for example, required local initiatives to meet the necessary educational requirements. The establishment of a new clinical department often requires extensive manipulation of available staff and facilities. The person at General Hospital who has been most successful in carrying out fact-finding studies is the hospital director. His ability can be exemplified by the establishment of the department of orthopaedics—the decision to open this was partly the result of a campaign on the part of a department chief. The hospital board carried out an extensive study in collaboration with the county council building department. After a great deal of deliberation, which involved possible relocation of parts of various clinical departments, facilities for orthopaedics were temporarily arranged in the new long-term care unit. A permanent location was also provided in the multi-storey building then under construction.

In other instances, such as the introduction of medical check-ups, extensive studies were performed at General Hospital under the guidance of one or several department heads. Medical check-ups were undertaken on an experimental basis in 1965, and the findings used to evaluate the possibilities of providing this service on a larger scale.

Decisions on strategic changes are made exclusively by the county council, especially by the influential executive committee. On the other hand, interviews indicated that department chiefs—individually and as a group—were often highly influential and much more active than the trustees in forcing a decision. The trustees acted more in a scrutinising capacity, by conveying proposals, with the approval of the department chiefs, to the county council for decision. The National Board of Health and Welfare often has veto power over strategic planning, especially as it approves or rejects requests for new department chief positions. In 1965, the board also presented a formal request to be informed about plans to coordinate planning in various county councils, but this does not seem to have affected the way in which strategic planning is carried out at General Hospital.

We expected the management to consider strategic changes in order to solve personnel problems and try to 'limit the hospital's assortment'. This expectation was only partially realised. Our inventory of matters dealt

182

with by the trustees during 1964 and 1965 showed that these questions were seldom handled systematically. But interviews with members of the board indicated that they sometimes discussed personnel matters in principle, i.e. methods for recruiting nurses, male medical service personnel, age limits for employment, and reduction of the nurses' workload. Lessening the load on in-patient units by treating more people as outpatients provides one example of an issue that was discussed because of staff shortages, though it is also a strategic problem related to assortment.

According to the interviewees, the trustees' involvement in these matters was very limited owing to lack of time. The executive committee, however, was much more active, and proposed all the changes that can be regarded as strategic. Advertisements for Scandinavian physicians were published regularly, and often produced results. Advertisements in the German press led to employment of a number of German physiotherapists. The hospital director had informal contact with the National Board of Health and Welfare to discuss the possibility of recruiting Irish nurses. The chief nurse had similar contacts with this board with respect

TABLE 6.3

The hospital management's involvement in some strategic matters.

Matter discussed	By board of trustees	By department chief association
1 Possibility of recruiting foreign manpower on a large scale	No	No
2 Status of research and education of doctors at General Hospital	Yes, indirectly on occasion	Yes
3 Possibility of locating parts of General Hospital's activities abroad (such as long-term care of arthritic and rheumatic patients)	No	No
4 Measures which would radically change the division of labour between doctors and nurses at General Hospital	No	No
5 Possibility of collaborating to set up group practices, secondary hospitals, etc. in order to make General Hospital's function more distinct	No	Yes
6 Fundamental objectives of continued expansion at General Hospital	Yes	Yes
7 Balance between in-patient and outpatient care at General Hospital	Yes, to some extent	Yes

to recruiting foreign nurses. The subcommittee has also dealt with several important issues related to the reallocation of work among personnel groups. Examples include a new job as ward clerk to reduce nurses' desk work in various units,[4] replacement of junior doctors through deputy department chief appointments and, of course, all the matters mentioned previously in our inventory of the hospital board's work.

A similar review of the activities of the department chiefs' association in 1965 showed that department chiefs are more active than the board of trustees in these matters, and have taken more initiatives. The association appointed a group to study the work performed by social workers, occupational therapists, and physiotherapists. It also handled a proposal to set up a clinic for treatment of acute alcoholism.[5] A number of personnel matters were also discussed by the department chiefs' association. Table 6.3 contains an incomplete but more specific comparison of the board of trustees and department chief's association, and is based on a questionnaire and interviews.

The hospital management's role in participant administration

Expectations

Some expectations as to the importance of the hospital management in strategic planning were formulated and discussed in the preceding section. We found that the management's freedom of action and resources were very limited in this context. With respect to the description of the hospital's relations to its participants (see chapter 4), and particularly, the difficult problem of satisfying the demands of certain participants, we might expect the management to be highly active when it comes to formulating policy. But certain factors imply that the contrary is more likely. Leaving matters to the county council, complex triangular relations, and lack of sanctions against some participants all indicate that the hospital's management might have to retreat—not only in terms of strategic planning but also in matters related to policy formulation. This implies that the county council can be expected to have assumed the role of policy maker.

Measurements

This section describes the way in which different subpolicies, such as personnel, patient, and public relations policies, are formulated. We tried

184

to evaluate the importance of the hospital's management in formulating policy by making a list of as many recent significant policy matters as possible and by studying how the management affected the policy which emerged. Our method consisted primarily of an informal 'search' throughout our study of the hospital and resulted in a list which included the following:

Distribution of housing among different personnel groups.
Scheduling of on-call duty service.
Allocation of long-term care resources among different patient groups.
Allocation of the resources of different clinical departments among in-patients and patients on the waiting list.
Objectives for the activities of new clinical departments.
Balancing purchases between the county council's central purchasing department and other suppliers.

For those who know something about a hospital's situation, this list gives a good idea of policy formulation within the hospital. There are a number of reasons why the hospital's management has almost completely withdrawn from policy making.

First, the most important group of policy matters—involving a confrontation of different demands for which resolution of conflict is required—has been referred to the doctors (via legislation) under the heading 'medical matters'. It is also obvious that a decision as to whether patient A or patient B is admitted from the waiting list, or patient C, who needs additional care, requires medical expertise. But the doctors' influence and responsibility are not limited to factual evaluations. Their opinions serve to a large extent as the basis for formulated priorities, for instance, in decisions to discharge or admit patients, to grant requests for abortions, etc.

These matters are particularly relevant when new specialities are to be established in Industry Town, i.e. long-term care, orthopaedics, and child psychiatry. The county council was especially interested in how resources allotted to the chronic diseases unit would be used, and even presented the department head with some guidelines. But it should be noted that the department head believed that he had the final responsibility, and did not act in accordance with the council's proposals in all instances. One of the department heads involved complained about the difficulty of obtaining fundamental decisions as to the construction, resources, and objectives of the unit.

185

The hospital's management has also refrained from formulating policy in other instances. Often, it has simply left policy formulation to others who are in a position to take a stand, and able to find solutions. One example of this is in purchasing policy. Another example concerns the way in which the on-call duty of doctors has been discussed and handled at the hospital. A doctor on call is responsible for care of the acutely ill outside regular working hours, i.e. he takes care of acute cases that come to the hospital requesting care, and steps in when hospitalised patients present acute symptoms or complications at night or on weekends. On-call duty is traditionally allocated among the doctors so that each department has one doctor on call—usually a junior who is always at the hospital— and a back-up physician—usually a department head who can be called to the hospital if the younger doctor thinks he needs help. On-call duty has always been particularly burdensome and disliked by the younger doctors. This service also constitutes an area in which different groups of doctors have had conflicting interests. These conflicting interests involve not only the junior v. the senior doctors, but also the 'heavy' v. the 'light' departments. The medical, surgical, and obstetrical departments have a large number of emergencies, while certain others have a much smaller number.

We had an opportunity to study how conflicts were resolved and policies formulated in two special instances at General Hospital. The first concerned distribution of the on-call workload between the departments of medicine and psychiatry. The principal issue was the way in which doctors from these departments took care of emergencies involving certain types of poisoning (alcohol, narcotics, etc.). The psychiatrists had repeatedly refused to serve on an on-call basis because they said they were understaffed. After long discussions between the junior doctors in these departments—in which department heads and the hospital management neither participated nor took sides—an agreement was reached. Doctors in the department of psychiatry would not have to be on call, but at 8 a.m. were to assume responsibility for all emergencies requiring psychiatric treatment. This agreement was confirmed in a formal contract, signed by two junior doctors and approved by the heads of the two departments.

The second example had to do with on-call compensation for junior doctors. The county council central wages board and the Swedish Medical Association negotiated a pay agreement which took effect on 1 January 1962. The Medical Association demanded compensation for doctors required to be on call. But a valid agreement was not reached until two years later. Beginning in September 1964, doctors on call would receive either extra vacation days or monetary compensation corresponding to the number of hours on duty. This agreement initiated a number of ques-

186

tions in all hospitals with regard to the organisation of on-call service and compensation. The parties to the agreement appointed a coordinating committee which included a Member of Parliament, a department chief, a management consultant from the Association of County Councils, a hospital director, and two associate members (a young doctor and an employee of the Swedish Young Physicians' Association). What interested us most in this context was not the uncertainty caused by the agreement, nor the solutions specific to General Hospital, but the way in which decisions of this kind are reached at General Hospital. But first, we shall include a description of the decision-making process within the hospital as perceived by the coordinating committee:

In administrative matters, the hospital adheres to the same rules for delegation of authority and responsibility as does any public legal subject. This means that the board of trustees has the right of decision in all matters. Certain tasks are expressly assigned to a higher authority, in this case the county Health and Medical Services Board. Other responsibilities have been delegated to employees of the hospital's management through directives based on health and medical care legislation and ordinances. This applies, for example, to the director responsible for ensuring that on-call duty is satisfactorily regulated. However, neither the director nor the physician (department chief) has any independent right of decision. Even though the latter is also assigned certain specific tasks, both are obliged to adhere to the decisions of the board of trustees.

One important exception concerned the department chiefs, who do not come under the trustees' jurisdiction in matters which could be 'directly related to medical activities'. The hospital legislation committee expressed this as follows in a report from 1956 (Swedish Government Official Reports 1956:27): 'It has been deemed suitable to clearly express the fact that physicians' medical activities do not come under the jurisdiction of the local hospital's management, the Board of Trustees or the Medical Services Board, while the physicians do not assume any special position in an administrative sense in relation to other authorities. The physicians have to adhere to what these authorities prescribe, obviously provided that these directives do not involve any conflict with rules and regulations established by hospital legislation and ordinances.'

Thus, the question arises as to whether or not decisions regarding on-call duty should be classified as medical activity. The legislators have instructed the director to be responsible for a satisfactory

187

on-call system. If this section of the law is to have any significance, this has to mean that, in a conflict between the director and the department chief in question, the director must have the right to decide in matters of this kind since he is the responsible authority. This, in turn, implies that the director's decision can be superseded by a board decision, since the director is not in an independent position; he is dependent on the superior authority, whose right of decision in certain matters has only been delegated to him. This interpretation implies that matters related to on-call duty have been removed from the group of tasks for which the physician has the exclusive right of decision.

The actual decision-making process was quite different, however. 'Diary notes' on this matter, beginning in March 1964, when the problem of compensation for on-call service was dealt with by the hospital board of trustees, included the following: The chief of the medical staff was asked to find a solution. This was followed by discussions in the department chiefs' association, and negotiations between representatives of the junior doctors and the board. A solution was finally arrived at in January 1965, whereby extra doctors were recruited to ensure that compensatory time off could be taken. But problems with respect to on-call service still remained, and were acute in some instances. Meetings again took place, in 1965, involving the department chiefs' association, the hospital's executive committee, the board of trustees, and the junior doctors. These meetings resulted in a proposal for on-call compensation which was agreed to by all parties.[6]

The overall picture with respect to these two examples is fairly simple. Policy formulation was achieved through negotiations between the groups involved, i.e. the senior and junior doctors. The hospital's board of trustees, through the hospital director, intervenes only when the situation becomes deadlocked.

Before we summarise and give our interpretations, we turn to an example which is an exception to the general rule that the hospital management refrains from formulating policy. The situation involved a conflict between different participants in which the management clearly took sides. The problem was whether or not to close an in-patient unit. As usual, the cause was a staff shortage which made it impossible to assign enough nurses to the unit. The charge nurse said that she 'couldn't cope any longer' and requested that the unit be closed. The supervisory and chief nurses supported her in their loyalty towards the staff, i.e. overwork

188

would certainly reduce the amount of staff even further. But the department head felt that the unit should remain open because of a long waiting list, including many serious cases. The hospital director decided in favour of the department head, and thus managed to keep the unit open for the time being.

But, in general, the hospital management does not think that it has an obligation, or even the ability, to reconsider the hospital's strategy, which is more or less given 'from above'. Privately, members of the management may believe that it is wrong, for instance, to allot such a large portion of the hospital's resources to outpatient care. But, in their capacities as trustee or hospital director, they have little opportunity for influencing conditions, and have to remain loyal to the guidelines prescribed by higher authorities. Policy formulation, i.e. creating rules for handling different participants, or resolving conflicts between them, is not suited to the activities of the hospital management. Relations with each participant group can be solved as isolated subproblems. As opposed to industrial firms, the hospital does not have to balance the interests of customers against those of personnel and owners. The most important problem of priorities is related to the balance between different groups of patients and individuals who make claims on the scarce resources of the hospital. This, and other policy matters, are usually solved by professional groups, primarily by contact with colleagues outside the hospital. The hospital's purchasers collaborate with those in the county council who negotiate bulk and other purchases. The hospital director has tried to establish working contact with directors of some nearby hospitals, mainly to establish a common staff policy. The recently appointed personnel manager is a member of a personnel manager association.

But medical policy matters create the most extensive problems, which are discussed primarily by the professional corps. Debate between doctors takes place through the medical journals, at various medical conventions, international conferences, and at the hospital itself (in their Saturday staff meeting). Medical and technical matters are usually discussed at the staff meeting, though a few younger department heads have tried to call attention to policy matters.

Planning for resource procurement

Expectations

The hospital's need to expand and its relatively good opportunities for

189

predicting the long-term development of demand for medical services not only require, but also facilitate long-term planning of expansion. One of the consequences of this activity is the need for long-term planning for resource procurement.

We expected this planning to be aimed at coordinating the supply of personnel, financing, and procurement of material resources such as buildings and other technical equipment. These three types of resources are the most difficult to obtain, and one of them can always be expected to be scarce at any given time. In addition, the hospital does not have a great deal of automation, i.e. machines are, more or less, merely tools. Thus, expansion of the production apparatus depends on the supply of qualified personnel. Long-term investment planning, in light of a shortage of staff, has to be coordinated with planning for recruitment and education. We expected the time required for resource procurement to be a minimum of five years.

Measurements

Our impression of how the hospital plans resource procurement is based on studies of available plans, and interviews with the individuals involved in planning. This means that we interviewed about ten people at the hospital and in the county council.

Early each spring, the hospital drafts its general and salary budgets. The proposals are drafted by those responsible for the various clinical departments. After informal consultation with the department chief association, the drafts are presented to the trustees. Requests for financial and personnel resources are coordinated with those of the administration and other departments. The trustees devote about an hour to this matter, but, prior to this, the budgets have been checked by the hospital director and the executive committee. The budgets are then processed by various agencies of the county council. Table 6.4 shows how budget processing involves successive bargaining and reductions. Corresponding examples for 1965 were given in chapter 4.

None of the seventeen specialties, nor the hospital as a whole, has any formally written long-term plan for resource requirements or procurement. But several department chiefs, and the hospital's management, do claim to have specific ideas about the amount of resources they intend to request during the next few years. They also have definite opinions as to the most urgent areas of expansion.

A so-called five-year plan is drawn up by the county council, and in-

190

cludes forecasts of resources required by the various sectors of county activity. General Hospital is not listed separately, however. The county council handles the plan internally, and the hospital is not consulted, mainly because the general plan is intended as a rough liquidity statement.

County council planning also includes a long-term investment plan. The most recent was formulated in 1953 and is no longer valid. It is now being revised. In contrast to our expectations, this plan only covers approximate cost estimates; no real quantitative plan and no evaluations of personnel requirements or supply are included. When we asked about the reasons for these findings, we encountered a kind of doomsday philosophy: 'We know it's going to be hard to recruit staff—but all the county councils are in the same boat and plan the same way we do. Anyway, we won't have more problems than anybody else.' Others are highly critical because this type of planning has to be based on available personnel resources. They readily point out that, during the past five years, five fully equipped nursing units had to remain closed owing to lack of personnel and that the newly built department of psychiatry could open only three of its units.

Personnel administration

Expectations

The hospital's difficulty in acquiring and satisfying the demands of personnel makes staff administration one of the most important tasks of hospital management. We expected the hospital to have extensive personnel services with several well-qualified employees wholly or partly devoted to personnel matters. On the basis of comparisons with Swedish industrial firms, we estimated that from five to eight full-time employees would be required for the personnel department.

The division of the hospital into fairly small, autonomous subsystems requires informal administrative contacts. An extensive division into highly self-confident professional groups makes it difficult for anyone who is not a professional to handle certain personnel administrative matters. We expected much of the personnel administrative work and decision making to be decentralised. We also expected many department chiefs to be involved in personnel matters, though inconsistencies between their interests would tend to create wide differences between departments. But the strong personnel organisations found in the national trade unions, and the considerable size of the hospital, also led us to expect a central personnel service of high status. This service would create common

191

TABLE 6.4
Budget processing, 1966

Date	Discussed by	Action	Approximate no. of working hours	Decision 1966 expressed as % of decision 1965		Most important support motive
				Operating budget	Capital budget	
January-February	Department and unit chiefs	Proposed request drafted	3-15 hours/unit			Increasing load; medical and technical development; possibility of reducing amount of personnel
February	Department chiefs' association	Informal discussion of requests made by the different departments	3-hour meeting	No significant changes in original proposals		Coordination of requirements
February	Department and unit chiefs	Request presented to trustees		Cannot be estimated in % since these requests are often not expressed in cr. or in some other specific calculable way		See above
March	Hospital director, chief accountant and personnel dept.	Preparation	3-5 weeks	See above		Review of cost estimates, feasibility, and urgency
March	Executive committee	Discussion of difficult factual matters	2-3 meetings of 4 hours each			Review of feasibility and urgency
March-April	Board of trustees	Report—no real factual discussion	1 hour meeting	120%	125%	

192

Table 6.4 (continued)

April-May	County council office		Approx. 1 man-week	Formal scrutiny; review of cost estimates; coordination of measures at other hospitals in the county
June	Direct contacts between executives in the county council	Discussion of 'unclear' issues	1 day meeting in Industry Town	See above
June	Health and medical services board (augmented by medical representatives for in-patient care in the county)	Report–short discussion	1 hour during a meeting	
September	Executive committee	Approval of the county council budget in its entirety	5 minutes during a meeting	119% 121%
October	County council	Confirmation	5 minutes in committee	

guidelines, see to it that agreements and instructions were observed, provide the departments with support, and if individual departments were not interested in personnel matters, compensate for this lack of interest.

Owing to the acute personnel problems, we expected the most important aspects of personnel administrative work performed in the clinical departments and central personnel department to be concerned with short-term matters. Recruitment, introduction, salaries, benefits, disputes, and complaints would be the most typical and time consuming. Especially in the central personnel department, we expected to find planned or executed measures aimed at releasing resources for education and long-term reduction of staff turnover.

We also thought that personnel problems would lead to discussions and experiments in new forms of cooperation with employees. We expected to find experiments in progress such as appointment of representatives from different personnel groups to the board of trustees, direct cooperation between the hospital's management and the unions, and extension of the employee-management committee. On the other hand, the autonomy of the various units could be expected to imply successful cooperation with employees at the department level, i.e. most matters significant to the employees can be solved on this level. Another incentive for efforts to alter cooperative institutions was related to our expectations that the management would regard as serious problems such factors as the high degree of professional differentiation involving several unions, varying salary systems, and competition between professional groups.

We also had expectations as to personnel policy. Powerful trade unions and difficulty in satisfying demands of the personnel should create a strong need for definite personnel policies. Personnel policy is required as an instrument for influencing the expectations of the staff and for ensuring consistent supervisory behaviour. This implies that personnel policy should primarily handle matters regarded as vital to personnel loyalty and turnover, i.e. salaries, housing, education, and promotion. Membership of a larger organisation (the county council) and an employer association (the Association of County Councils) implies that the hospital's policy has to be coordinated within the guidelines of larger organisations. But extreme differences between the departments, in terms of size and autonomy, sometimes lessen the value of a uniform policy. This could also mean that fixed guidelines might be interpreted as bureaucracy and an obstacle to flexibility in personnel management.

Low predictability, large variations in workload, and the power of the personnel probably imply that staff at the hospital are sometimes deployed ineffectively. But the demand for efficiency is not particularly

194

great. Thus, we expected that controls on slack would be assigned little importance. Differences in technology and workloads between departments and other units would also tend to make the problem of organisational slack vary from one department to the next. This condition combined with the low level of automation made us expect that controls on slack would be carried out by persons in supervisory positions.

Measurements

People at the hospital are well aware of the importance of personnel matters. Vacancies, closed nursing units, and unqualified temporary staff are constant reminders of staff problems that cannot be avoided. All our interviews quickly got around to personnel matters. People in supervisory positions often said that personnel problems were not only a question of recruitment. New demands from employees over matters such as fixed working hours make it increasingly difficult to make effective use of staff who, in turn, are less and less willing to accept inconvenient working hours, or transfers from one place of work or task to another.

Personnel service at the hospital is well established in one respect. The board of trustees devotes, on average, 20 per cent of its meetings to personnel matters. The executive committee spends even more time handling these affairs. In addition, the county Health and Medical Service Board devotes about 50 per cent of its meetings to staff matters.

In accordance with a request from the county council, the hospital has also commissioned a firm of management consultants to study the organisation of the personnel department. After this survey was completed, two teams led by department chiefs continued the study. As a result, some personnel administrative routines were surveyed, and various aspects of personnel policy reviewed. Recent decisions by the executive committee of the county council have resulted in the establishment of several new positions in the personnel department. Unfortunately, some of these remain unfilled. The new organisation of the personnel department, together with personnel resources, as compared with those of four years earlier are shown in Figure 6.1.

In contrast to our expectations, most of the personnel administrative routines at the hospital appeared to be extremely formal, and the authority to make decisions was—formally at least—generally very centralised. This is partly because existing public health laws and collective agreements allow the county council to exert a great deal of control, particularly through the executive committee's wages board (see chapter 4; in parti-

195

cular Table 4.4). Since the wages board has the final word in salary matters, the hospital management automatically becomes involved in the preparation and presentation of each case to go before the board. The hospital director is often called on to act as personnel manager since this position is vacant for the time being. Employees in the personnel department provide information and investigate the various matters requiring decisions. Table 6.5 indicates some examples of the decision-making process for the most usual types of personnel matters.

However, the real decisions on personnel matters are made primarily on two levels. The Association of County Councils, i.e. the central employer organisation, regulates all matters concerning working time, benefits, and other employment conditions, through collective agreements with about twenty employee organisations. The hospital and the county councils often try to circumvent these agreements. For instance, they might make a generous interpretation of regulations on the number of years' service to be credited, travel expenses, etc. But these possibilities are limited. Within the framework of agreements, decisions on selection of applicants for employment, length of holidays, etc. are made at a fairly low level and, to a large extent, by heads of departments and supervisory nurses. Thus, differences between the real decision-making process and formal decision authority are sometimes a source of conflict, e.g. when a department chief's promise to an employee is, for some reason, not respected by the central authorities.

This centralisation of personnel decisions may be one reason why heads of departments, and others in positions of authority, usually seem to feel little responsibility for personnel welfare. In any case, the systematised, more informal personnel welfare measures reported are not very extensive (see Table 6.6).

The status of the employees in the personnel department, and even that of the currently vacant position of personnel manager, is uncertain and controversial. The newly appointed personnel officers have more or less to 'fight for existence'. The tasks of the new personnel department include some phases of the hiring process, such as contacts with the national employment agency and job applicants. These regulations are often circumvented, questioned, and criticised at General Hospital, and there is also a great deal of dissatisfaction with the personnel department's way of handling various matters. These are all signs of the unclear status of the personnel department and its employees. The board of trustees proposed that the personnel manager should be placed somewhere between salary grades KA 21 and KA 25. The county council's executive committee, however, thought that salary grade KA 21 would suffice.[7] We studied

196

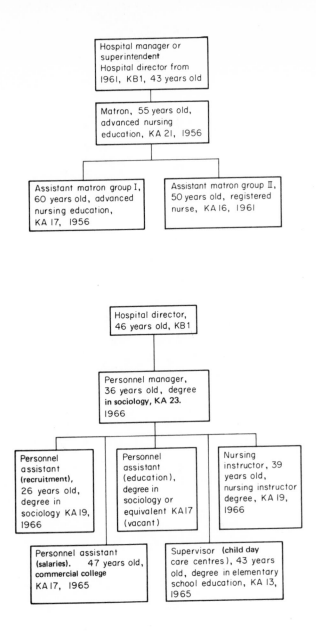

Fig. 6.1 Organisation and employees in the personnel department at General Hospital before and after 1966 (KA and KB refer to salary grades; see chapter 4).

TABLE 6.5

The formal decision-making process for some routine personal matters

Subject	Phase in the decision-making process		
	Initiative	Preparation	Decision
Appointment of department chief	Board of trustees	Personnel department, National Board of Health and Welfare, department chiefs' association, board of trustees	Swedish Government
Employment of full-time junior doctor	Head of the clinical department	County council's expert on merits and qualifications, department chief, personnel department, board of trustees	Swedish Government
Employment of full-time nurse	Supervisory nurse or department chief	Initiator, personnel department, employment agency	Board of trustees
Employment of assistant nurse or nursing auxiliary	Supervisory nurse	Personnel department, supervisory nurse, work supervisor (usually charge nurse)	Board of trustees
Employment of maids	Chief of maintenance	Personnel department, (chief of maintenance)	Board of trustees
Employment of locum doctor	Department chief or person appointed by him (such as assistant department chief)	Initiator	Department chief
Employment of temporary nursing substitute	Supervisory nurse	Specially appointed 'recruiter of temporary staff' in personnel department	'Recruiter' and supervisory nurse
Salary grade promotion not stipulated in collective bargaining agreements	Employee or his/her boss	Supervisor involved, personnel department and/or hospital director, board of trustees	Executive committee's wages board

198

Table 6.5 (continued)

Granting of leave of absence (less than three months)	Employee	Heads of departments involved, personnel department	Board of trustees
Granting of leave of absence (more than three months)	Employee	Heads of departments involved, personnel department, hospital director	Executive committee's wages board
Granting doctors' holiday time	Department chief	Department chief or his assistant, usually another physician	Board of trustees
Granting vacation time for other medical service personnel	Supervisory and chief nurses	Department chief, supervisory and chief nurses, personnel department	Personnel department
Assignment of staff housing or priority on municipal housing waiting lists	Employee	Personnel department, hospital director	Board of trustees
Granting of travel expenses for educational trips	Employee	Heads of departments involved, personnel department, board of trustees	Executive committee's wages board

199

wage statistics from the National Employers' Association which, surprisingly, showed large variations in the distribution of wages. This reflects the fact that the status of personnel managers in private industry is also unclear. Despite this reservation, and the knowledge that government positions usually command less pay than corresponding jobs in industry, it will probably be very difficult to find a qualified person for the job of personnel manager at the salary level indicated by the executive committee.

One of our expectations was fully realised, that short-term personnel tasks predominated at General Hospital. Employment matters, hiring of substitutes, solving housing problems for new employees and temporary staff, planning the holiday rota, calculation of holiday pay, setting up new personnel budgets, distributing much sought-after places in child day-care centres, and other similar problems, large and small, all tend to keep the understaffed personnel department, nursing supervisors and, often, even department chiefs busy. These tasks have gradually been concentrated in the new personnel department. But all heads of departments still feel directly or indirectly (e.g. through the deputy department

TABLE 6.6

Informal personnel welfare measures at General Hospital.

Which of the following personnel welfare measures have you applied in your department or unit?

a staff parties b trips, study visits, etc. c information meetings	Daily	Weekly	Monthly	Quarterly	Annually	Rarely	Never	No answer	Not applicable
Clinical departments									
Department chiefs' answers									
a					7	1	5	2	1
b			1		2	4	6	2	1
c	2	3	1	1	1	5	2		1
Nursing units									
Charge nurses' answers									
a				1	6	5	4		
b						3	11	1	1
c	1	1	4	2		5	2		1

200

chiefs) responsible for hiring locums and reallocating personnel when opening or closing a unit.

Since wage and benefit matters have been centralised in the county council's wages board, the personnel department does not have to allot much time to these items. Time-consuming investigations in doubtful cases are seldom necessary, especially as the personnel department does not have the authority to make decisions anyway. Matters such as these are immediately referred to the wages board.

The emphasis on short-term tasks is also supported by the almost complete absence of long-term development projects in the personnel area. There are a few, however. Two groups chaired by department chiefs are working with the management consultants mentioned earlier to investigate recruiting and internal personnel routines. So far, this work has been carried out parallel with normal personnel service. The most important project in the personnel department involves updating the personnel register, which has previously existed mainly in the memories of various persons and in certain private files.

Our expectations that personnel problems would lead to experiments in new forms of cooperation were only partly realised. The forms of cooperation now in use were described in chapter 4. The most important considerations have had to do with market contact. Personnel specialists want more active contacts with potential employees, e.g. through information for potential nursing students and advertisements in other counties and abroad. Measures aimed at more active competition for personnel with other hospitals in the county, or in other counties, are obstructed to a large extent by the national employment agency which tries to prevent 'excessively active' personnel recruitment. It is difficult to begin considering a change in the institutions for negotiating with employee organisations since conditions depend on central agreements and the way in which they are written.

Table 6.7 shows that the employee-management committee at General Hospital functions in roughly the same way as most, similar committees in industrial firms. The hospital management does not feel the committee is very meaningful so far as personnel administration is concerned. An extension of the activities of the employee-management committee, and the establishment of rules for departmental and unit meetings, have been contemplated but not put into effect. On the other hand, no consideration has been given to the idea of including personnel groups other than department chiefs in board of trustees meetings. Department chiefs are present at board meetings in their capacity as heads of clinical departments, not as employees.

201

The hospital does not have any written personnel policy. But through agreements with employee organisations (a total of almost thirty agreements) wages and indirect benefits and matters such as recruitment and promotion are regulated. The county council and its wages board have also made statements of principle and established definite practices and precedents in many matters, such as the important area of education. The hospital is very generous in this field, and, in principle, grants loans or scholarships for further education. The best example of educating personnel at the expense of the hospital is that nursing auxiliaries can be trained to become assistant nurses; there are also other cases, e.g. the education of nurses, doctors, personnel and other assistants. Employees can receive support in these and many other areas according to recommendations from the Association of County Councils. In connection with the management consultants' study of the hospital's personnel administration, the board was advised by the consultants to formulate certain goals for personnel policy (see Table 6.8). There is not yet a complete set of principles for handling personnel administrative matters but work is in progress to establish one.

Our expectation that people in some units or clinical departments would be highly critical of personnel policy was only partly met. However, our method of measurement in this instance may have been unsatisfactory. Table 6.9 shows that, even though a fairly large number of people are critical, many others have a very positive attitude towards the hospital's personnel policy. Some supervisors are more positive towards personnel policy than are the department chiefs. We were unable to find a systematic relation between the size or autonomy of a clinical department and its attitudes towards personnel policy. But there is some relation between the attitudes of supervisors and their involvement in personnel welfare (measured in terms of their own statements and evaluations of the five people at General Hospital whom we thought had the best perspective). On the whole, we believe that the attitudes reflected in Table 6.9 do not deviate much from what can be expected in an industrial firm.

The most important kind of slack in organisations is revealed when an organisation's resources are used by its members for private purposes, so that it becomes overstaffed, and the employees underutilised. Therefore, we studied the controls on slack used to counteract these two phenomena.

We tried to find out the extent to which the hospital's resources are used for private purposes by making informal interviews whenever we had an opportunity to broach such a sensitive subject. We believe that the picture we finally obtained is both plausible and reasonable. The resource which can be regarded as being used for private purposes is the doctors' time—

TABLE 6.7

Matters dealt with by the employee-management committee during 1965.

Meeting no. 1
1 New member
2 Centralised cleaning
3 Library committee to handle professional literature for personnel
4 New child day-care centre
5 Courses
6 Member of suggestion committee
7 Proposal from an employee about shock absorbers for scooters
8 Proposal from supervisory nurse about using the central radio system
   for daily personnel information

Meeting no. 2
9 Newspapers for personnel
10 'Day-care centre' contest
11 Proposals for saving supplies
12 Autumn courses, 1965
13 Report from the staff club

Meeting no. 3
14 Disappearance of white coats
15 Pay day for monthly wages
16 Leisure activities during 1965
17 Utilisation of male personnel in nursing care
18 Information from the Swedish Council for Personnel Administration
    about personnel matters
19 New child day-care centre
20 Course in personnel management
21 Proposals for rewards

Meeting no. 4
22 Composition of the employee-management committee
23 Proposal for an 'improved' workbench
24 Report on the personnel situation
25 Staff party

TABLE 6.8

Proposals for personnel policies at General Hospital

The personnel policy that the board of trustees wants to put into effect is aimed at:

1 Creating a spirit of confidence and cooperation at the hospital, to give employees a feeling of security and belonging
2 Attaining efficiency and well-being via modern management
3 Through close cooperation with the hospital's personnel organisations, arriving at solutions to mutual problems that are satisfactory to all concerned
4 Acquiring good employees through active recruiting and hiring procedures and modern personnel planning
5 Taking care of new employees, through a well-planned induction course, in order to give them a good start at the hospital, and following a similar course when introducing existing employees to new duties
6 Providing employees with opportunities for further education
7 Stimulating the employee-management committee and suggesting activities to work actively
8 Providing information about the hospital and its activities via thorough and detailed internal and external information
9 Facilitating the adjustment of employees to their working environment, and vice versa, by means of an effective personnel service

to the extent that it is used for outpatient care or for research, thus giving doctors income, acclaim, etc. Doctors have complete control over resources because of the way in which jobs are allocated within the clinical departments. The department chief decides how much time a junior doctor can devote to outpatient care, or the amount of resources to be allotted to a research project. (The extent of research was described in chapter 5.) Department chiefs in many specialties think that junior doctors should be allowed to earn extra income from outpatient care—otherwise they would not be able to recruit junior doctors. Our interviews also revealed that the service personnel who have to assist the doctors sometimes regarded research as inconvenient, extra work.

Secretaries are another 'resource' available to those in authority, even for tasks not directly related to the working situation. But in this instance, the hospital's norms seem to be much more severe than an industrial firm's. A medical secretary should be used for medical work and, in most

204

cases, it is unthinkable that she be asked to plan a trip, arrange a purchase, or handle 'semi-private correspondence'. This is probably partly because norms in this area are generally much more stringent in public administration than in private firms, and the shortage of secretaries makes it difficult to accomplish even the medical work required. It may also arise through efforts at the hospital to make a clear distinction between an individual's professional and private roles. Thus, a secretary can only assist the doctor in his professional role and not as a private person.

Travel and entertainment expenses are carefully controlled. A study trip cannot be made without prior permission from the county council's wages board. On the other hand, travel expense accounts are not scrutinised as closely as they are in most industrial firms and government agencies. Entertainment accounts are small and dictated by norms set up by the county council. The general rule is that 'when entertainment, paying respects, etc. on behalf of the county council or its institutions is paid for by tax money, these kind of activities have to be kept within strict limits'.

TABLE 6.9

Attitudes of those in positions of authority towards personnel policy at General Hospital

There are some general rules at General Hospital with regard to the treatment of personnel

These rules:	Department chiefs	Charge nurses	Other supervisors
facilitate work to a large extent	2	6	2
facilitate work to some extent	3	12	9
do not mean very much	4	16	5
make work more difficult to some extent	4	3	2
make work more difficult to a large extent	1	1	0
No. of opinions	2	6	1
No. of respondents	16	44	19

A number of controls have been established at the hospital to prevent unnecessary or unsuitable use or purchase of supplies. These controls are more or less the same as those in industrial firms, though the hospital has not formulated any systematic methods such as value analysis. The most important controls are as follows. Purchases can be made only by a central purchasing office; the pharmacy at the hospital is responsible for the purchase and stocking of pharmaceuticals; supplies are kept in a central supply unit. Standardisation of many different kinds of supplies has been carried out centrally, but the pharmaceuticals committee at General Hospital has also considered an internal standardisation. The cost of pharmaceuticals and other supplies is supervised through a comparison of costs in different years. These comparisons are used as a basis for special studies of items such as the cost of X-ray film, certain disposable products, etc. Special conferences between the chief nurse and the nursing supervisors are held to discuss the testing of certain purchases.

Control of the number of employees in the clinical departments is based on various standards, which indicate the number of doctors, nurses, aides, medical secretaries, etc. which a unit is allowed in relation to a stipulated criterion, e.g. the number of patient days, number of patients, number of doctors etc. Some of these standards have been set up by the central public health authorities. The National Board of Health and Welfare also directly controls the number of doctors since new appointments cannot be made without its approval. In other cases, standards are based on studies carried out by the Association of County Councils, or obtained from informal comparisons of different hospitals and county council areas. One result of the standards system that we observed fairly often was that those in authority use these comparative figures as arguments in favour of their need to increase personnel. 'We're entitled to one more secretary.' 'I really (i.e., according to the National Board of Health and Welfare) should have one more junior doctor in my department but we've managed so far.'

The chief nurse and nursing supervisors are responsible for controlling the number of nurses and other medical service personnel. They also work with the special studies secretary in this matter. Special problems arise due to organisational or technological changes which allow for, or require, changes in the number of employees. This has occurred at General Hospital in connection with the introduction of central kitchen and cleaning services which allow a reduction of personnel in in-patients units. The county council also controls the number of employees in these instances via its organisation department. This latter type of control often implies that the hospital management, and sometimes the chief nurse, find them-

206

selves in conflicts where pressure is exerted from two different directions —one side exerting demands to reduce personnel, the other wanting to retain or increase staff. In each of the three cases that we were able to study, the chief nurse wholly or partially supported the clinical departments' demands for personnel, as opposed to 'the rationalisation authorities' requests for a staff reduction. The position of the hospital management was less clear.

Checks on the numbers of personnel through time and motion studies cannot be carried out to any large extent by the hospital itself, mainly because of a shortage of resources which can be allotted to such studies.

Attendance and punctuality are controlled by each department chief. This is done indirectly by the chief involved 'when he looks for or needs someone and discovers that his subordinate is there or is on time'. Most employees have a working schedule, and the need for cooperation is so great that this serves to control attendance and punctuality. Ten persons in supervisory positions who were interviewed on this matter said that they did not regard absenteeism and lateness as a problem. They claimed that employees found their jobs very stimulating and were loyal to their work and to General Hospital. The cases mentioned by more than one interviewee had to do with social workers, office staff and, especially, physiotherapists ('we never know where they are', 'they sit home drinking tea instead of going to the hospital'). But the only real conclusion that can be drawn from these interviews is that the problem is not regarded as severe. On the other hand, informal discussions indicated that many people thought that coffee breaks 'in certain departments and units were numerous and long'. The individual whom we judged to have the best contact with daily schedules expressed himself very drastically: 'The risk of coffee poisoning is much greater in many areas than the risk of overwork.' We did not observe any measures on the part of the hospital management, or others in supervisory positions, to control or reduce coffee breaks. Nor have coffee breaks been discussed by the board of trustees. They are regarded as legitimate, and a questionnaire to department chiefs, charge nurses, and others in supervisory positions revealed that everyone(!) took daily coffee breaks. Several persons—including department chiefs—stressed the importance of coffee breaks for informal conferences.

207

Patient administration

Expectations

It is very difficult for the hospital to satisfy patients' demands. There are conflicts of interest between different patient groups—if one group is satisfied, another has to be neglected—and between patients and other participants. Some examples are in patients' demands for on-call service v. physicians' demands for fixed working time, and patients demands for increased service v. taxpayers' demands for limits on county taxes. Resolution of conflicts such as these has to take place within the hospital, which, in turn, has to grade and often reject patients' demands. This is the main reason why we expected to find active efforts to influence patients' demands.

Another reason for this expectation is that large variations in workload, and the low predictability in production, make it difficult to achieve high efficiency in production. Therefore, the hospital should try—despite obvious difficulties—to get the 'right' patient to come to the hospital at the 'right' time. Since many of the hospital's difficulties stem from overloading, we also expected to find some kind of 'negative advertising', i.e. measures aimed at limiting demands for the hospital's services.

We had conflicting expectations as to the methods and organisation of patient administration. The high service content and the autonomy of units made us expect that the influence exerted on patients would be decentralised and involve almost all medical personnel. A great deal of responsibility should rest with the heads of the various units, i.e. with the heads of the clinical departments. But the difficulty in satisfying the demands of all patients and the public's demands for equal treatment made us expect that—despite decentralisation—the hospital would have centrally formulated policies governing its relations with patients. Thus, decentralised patient administration should be supported by measures and special resources from central authorities similar to those in other service agencies such as banks or restaurant chains.

Measurements

The results of our measurements of the hospital's resources and methods for patient administration are somewhat contradictory. Some of our observations indicate that the hospital has a great capacity for influencing patients and getting them to accept that some of their demands cannot be

208

met. On the other hand, we did not succeed in identifying the specialised resources and methods that we had thought were required.

A preliminary survey of the way in which the hospital receives the patient, and the methods used to influence demand, resulted in identification of four types of special patient administrative resources and measures:

1 Certain obstacles to the flow into the hospital.
2 Social workers whose task is to reduce demands for the hospital's service.
3 Some—though limited—information activity aimed at instructing patients how to behave at the hospital.
4 Medical check-ups.

There are three main obstacles: waiting lists, necessity for referral, and direct refusal to accept certain patient groups. The size of waiting lists was discussed in chapter 5. One important factor when it comes to understanding how the hospital functions is the influence which waiting lists have on demand. We did not have an opportunity to measure this relationship directly. Preliminary interviews indicated widely differing opinions. Some people thought waiting lists tended to reduce demand to some extent. Others felt that there were large groups of patients who actually liked waiting, and that a waiting list to get into the hospital was some kind of recommendation that tended to increase demand. A questionnaire sent

TABLE 6.10

Effects of waiting lists on the demand for hospital care

Do you feel that a waiting list and/or the amount of time spent in a waiting-room has some effect on keeping patients who do not require care away from the hospital?

| Response alternatives | Respondents (%) | | | | |
	Department chiefs	Other doctors	Charge nurses	Outpatient nurses	Other nurses
Yes, to a large extent	19	16	7	19	10
Yes, sometimes	31	40	21	38	30
No, hardly	18	37	21	38	43
No, just the opposite	25	2	0	6	2
No opinion/no answer	6	5	50	0	16
No. of respondents	16	38	43	16	61

to several personnel groups assumed to be in a position to evaluate this aspect revealed the same differences of opinion. The responses also showed that department heads in particular thought that waiting lists tended to increase demand. Of course, no reliable conclusions can be drawn about real conditions. It is possible that both opinions are correct. A waiting list of suitable length may increase demand, while an even longer waiting list may yield the opposite effect in another situation. One point that is certain on the basis of these 'contradictory opinions' is that the hospital does have the necessary knowledge to make systematic use of waiting lists to influence demand.

One clinical department and one assistant department chief at General Hospital work on a referral basis only. All other department chiefs say that they are against the referral requirement. Some even said—erroneously—that the prerequisite of a referral is not allowed. The reasons why doctors are against the referral requirement vary a great deal, as indicated by the following quotes (which include all the arguments given):

'Patients don't give up until they get a referral.' 'Some colleagues grant referrals which are based on doubtful indications.' 'It's important that a doctor examine each new case.' 'Doctors who make referrals are not specialists, so I have to evaluate whether or not the patient needs care anyway.' 'Relatives should also be able to have direct access to the hospital.' 'Free choice of doctor' (mentioned by four doctors). 'Unnecessarily complicated procedure from the patient's point of view.'

Junior doctors said that another important reason why some department chiefs were against referrals was that this tended to increase their workload, i.e. because the cases were more complicated. This, in turn, led to a decrease in personal (private) income. One department chief said that a referred case was usually twice as time consuming as a 'regular case', but that the pay was the same for each. The junior doctors in one department regularly had much higher incomes than the department chiefs because they were able to work with 'easier' outpatient cases.

Several department chiefs said that no patients who come to the hospital are turned away. In those instances when they go so far as to admit that this does occur, they claim that patients try to get priority on waiting lists without legitimate reasons (by coming to the clinic without an appointment, as an emergency case, etc.). Some patients are also turned away because they create a disturbance (not more than ten cases per year, say the department chiefs).

210

During one of our preliminary interviews, a social worker said that 'we really have to act as qualified bouncers—and that's not the way it's supposed to be'. Interviews with all the social workers, together with statistics on the social worker's tasks, were used to find out more about their influence on demand for the hospital's services. Those interviewed said that the social worker's main task (and that of her colleagues) was to assume responsibility for the often thankless and difficult job of finding post-hospital care: in convalescent homes, chronic hospitals, or even with relatives of the patient. These tasks predominate, for example, in the surgical, medical, and obstretrics and gynaecology departments. During 1965, the social worker in the medical, chest, and X-ray departments had contact with 478 patients; 257 of these contacts had to do with placement, and 216 were from the department of medicine. Social workers have similar tasks in the orthopaedic and rehabilitation departments, as in almost all others, with respect to helping patients return to work through contacts with various employers and vocational training agencies. The waiting list to the psychiatric department is the longest, and there is a social worker there whose main job is to screen the patient flow to the hospital. This social worker performs sociological studies which aid in grading the patients' priority. To some extent (if and when the patient can be admitted), these studies also serve as part of the basis for diagnosis and treatment. This social worker also said that her ability to give a patient direct support sometimes tended to make a visit to a doctor less urgent.

A booklet describing the hospital is given to every patient admitted for in-patient care, and information is also given by the charge nurse. One doctor has written an information booklet for a large group of patients; this aims mostly at reducing telephone inquiries. Various drug companies also supply a fairly large assortment of booklets for different groups of patients. But such booklets are used to a limited extent, and most of the doctors do not think that they are of much value. A few admitted that something might be gained by writing similar information booklets for even more groups of patients. Another of the social workers' tasks is to serve as a source of general information for patients. But they seldom take the initiative when it comes to providing information. Instead, they usually assume that patients in need of help will make the first contact.

Medical check-ups are also a means of influencing demand. They can be used to indicate that action should be taken at an early stage in an illness, at least so far as preventive measures are concerned. Check-ups also provide a means of examining a whole group of patients in a standard way.

Our preliminary interviews indicated that several department chiefs

211

were sceptical about the value of check-ups. The hospital management and the county council representative claimed that the hospital did not have resources for more extensive medical check-ups (see Table 6.11). The most interesting result of these interviews, from our point of view, was that none of those interviewed thought that check-ups were a means of freeing the hospital from a certain type of demand. Nor did they think that check-ups could increase the quality of the work performed at General Hospital.

Our expectation that most important decisions as to patients would be highly decentralised was, on the whole, fulfilled. Subordinates' opinions differed in many instances from those of the department chiefs as to who was responsible for patient administrative decisions. This points to differences between formal rules and the actual handling of these decisions.

But even if many decisions about satisfying patients' demands are made, for example, by the charge nurse, this usually occurs within a precise framework prescribed by the physician. Formulation of 'treatment policy', i.e. directives for treating patients, is obviously the task of the department chief or his assistant. This may refer to classifying patients on different kinds of waiting lists (see chapter 5), the duration of in-patient care (a social worker who understood our terminology used the expression 'bouncer policy'), the distribution of (often very sought-after) private rooms, permission to leave the hospital for short periods of time, etc.

We have to admit that it was extremely difficult to gain an understanding of the hospital's patient administration. Why do patients good-naturedly and patiently—almost without complaining, as we observed in chapter 5—sit in a waiting room for hours without any information about when their turn will come, or remain on waiting lists for weeks, and then come hours after they are summoned?

Obviously, the hospital has other and more adept methods of influencing patients (customers) than have oil companies or chain stores. The most important aspect here is that the doctors—owing to their status—have almost unlimited potential for influencing the patient. When we discussed this with various people at the hospital, we discovered similar opinions, though many thought these conditions were changing rapidly and that younger patients often regarded themselves, socially speaking, as the doctors' equal. But we did not attempt to measure these attitudes.

212

TABLE 6.11

Different types of medical check-ups which department chiefs thought should be performed during the next three years.[8]

Question to the department chiefs: 'What types of medical check-ups do you think should be performed at General Hospital during the *next three years* (under the auspices of the county council or in your specialty)?'

Previous check-ups that should be repeated during the next three years

Type of check-up and persons involved	Approx. no. of persons/year
Medical examination of 50 year-olds	2,000
Examination of all new-born infants	1,800
Examination of children (0-7 year-olds), child health clinic	4,000
Special examination of 4 year-olds	400
Chest X-rays of immigrants and others (heart and lungs — with X-ray contrast agent)	190,000
Gynaecological examination of women between 25 and 60	45,000
Laboratory test of uterine secretions from women born between 1920 and 1925	2,300
Chest X-rays of industrial and county employees	3,300

New check-ups that should be performed during the next three years

Type of check-up and persons involved	Approx. no. of persons/year
Gynaecological examination (cervix cancer test) of women between 30 and 60 years old (especially those between 40 and 50)	45,000
	2,000
Investigation of the incidence of diabetes in the county	240,000
Examination of urinary tract infections in all 50-year-old men and 30-year-old women	2,000
Review of all cases of mentally retarded children	800
Psychological examination of CP patients	
Examination of pre-school children (4 year-olds)	2,000-3,000
Investigation of the prevalence of phenylketonuria in all new-born infants	1,800
Simple pulmonary infections; all 40 year-olds	2,000
Clinical chemistry pilot study of all persons living in the county	240,000

Other participant administration and policies

Expectations

The hospital's strong position in relation to other participants made us expect that public relations would not be regarded as important as personnel and patient administration. But the hospital's importance in its geographical area in terms of employment and service, and the gradual growth of patient organisations, implied that some resources would be allotted to propagating information externally. Since the county council, the National Board of Health and Welfare, and the press seemed to be the most powerful participants, we expected this information activity to be directed primarily towards these three groups.

Measurements

Certain formally prescribed reporting channels are used for information to and from county authorities. The most important means are contacts between the board of trustees and the health and medical services board. All written communication is supposed to go through this channel. But matters involving wages have been delegated to others in the county council and the hospital. This means that there is a direct official channel between the personnel department and the county council's wages board. There is also official working contact between the accounts department at the hospital and the county council.

Informal contacts are usually made over the telephone. Visits are also made, at some level, an average of once a week. The daily mail regularly contains informal reports, excerpts from minutes, mimeographed reports, circulars, and other information from the county authorities to the hospital, and vice versa. These informal contacts can be regarded as taking place on four levels. The chairman of the board of trustees has informal contacts with the chairman of both the wages board and the health and medical services board. The hospital director has informal contacts with several of the top employees of the county council. At the expert level, the assistant from the wages board, the council's organisation assistant, and (when the budget is being worked on) the assistant in the county council finance department who is responsible for in-patient care, have repeated informal contacts with the hospital. The most frequent visitor to the hospital is the county council's organisation assistant (about twice a month). He believes that 'contacts will probably be even more frequent in

214

the future'. Another important contact is between the chairman of the county council and the department chiefs. 'Before General Hospital had a director, the department chiefs used to contact me directly and they've continued to do so. I know everyone doesn't like it but I think it's rather practical and I can't do much about it.' Contact channels are summarised in Table 6.12.

General Hospital provides the National Board of Health and Welfare with information through regular statistical reports and reports on specific matters, as necessary. A few department chiefs also have personal contact with members of the National Board of Health and Welfare. Information to municipal authorities is not very systematised. The chairman of the board of trustees, who has an important post in the municipal govern-

TABLE 6.12

General Hospital's contacts with the county authorities.

County authorities / Hospital	Executive committee and its chairman	Health and medical service board	County council chairman	Head of county council staff	County council wages board and its secretary	County council organisation assistant	County council assistant (in-patient care)	County council accounting department
Board of trustees and its chairman	Y	X			X			
Hospital director			Y	Y	X	Y	Y	
Chief of medical staff		Y	Y	Y	Y			
Assistant to the director						Y		
Chief nurse						Y		
Personnel department and its manager					X		Y	
Chief accountant						Y	Y	X
Department chief			Y					

X = channel used for official written information at least once a month
Y = channel used for informal contacts (written, telephone or visit) at least once a month

215

ment, handles all information over and above the daily contacts between the hospital and municipal employees.

The general information and press services (public relations department) at the hospital were more developed than we had expected. The hospital's management had been advised by experienced journalists when setting up its press service. This resulted in an organisation comparable with that of the most PR-oriented of industrial firms. The agenda and other information about meetings of the board of trustees are distributed to the local press in advance. This is done with confidence in the willingness of the press to regard the information as confidential until the meetings are over, but makes it easier for the press to contact the hospital's management for information about decisions made. Press conferences are held at intervals. Despite this central PR activity, there are no rules that forbid individuals to contact or provide information to the press —given, of course, general obligations to keep information about patients confidential. All department chiefs said that they have been in contact with the local press or national dailies on several occasions during the past few years. Two said that this kind of contact occurs nearly every week, or even more often. In exceptional cases, the department chiefs have been the ones to initiate a contact with the press. Many of the items refer to inquiries about accidents and patients treated. Medical news, newly opened departments and units, new equipment and medical research results also lead to contacts. One of the most common reasons for contact

TABLE 6.13

Attitudes towards active information at General Hospital

Do you think General Hospital should inform the general public about different medical and hospital matters through active contact with the press and in other ways?

Response alternatives (as %)	Respondents				
	Department chiefs	Deputy department chiefs and junior doctors	Charge nurses	Out patient nurses	Other nurses
Yes, definitely	25	42	17	13	26
Yes, possibly in certain matters	56	42	64	75	61
No, hardly	13	11	7	12	5
No, absolutely not	0	0	2	0	5
No opinion/no response	6	5	9	0	3
No. of respondents	16	38	44	16	61

216

with mass media is that a department chief is asked to give his opinion on matters currently being discussed in the national press.

In addition to giving information to the press, some department chiefs are fairly active in lecturing on current medical problems. Personnel at the hospital give about twenty lectures per year to various associations, schools, etc. Some doctors and nurses also participate in extensive teaching at the School of Nursing. Several department chiefs and the hospital director are members of the rotary club in Industry Town. An exhibit depicting the history of the hospital was on display at the hospital in the winter of 1965.

Our preliminary interviews as to the hospital's information activities revealed highly varying attitudes. Some thought that people at the hospital were much too passive in providing information. Others thought it wrong for a hospital actively to inform the press. When this was done, it led to misunderstandings, anxiety, etc. We tried to classify these attitudes more systematically through a questionnaire to doctors and nurses (Table 6.13).

Most of those in the groups questioned had positive attitudes towards General Hospital actively giving information to the press. The junior doctors were more categorically in favour of this activity than were department heads. It was more difficult to ascertain whether there were differences between groups of nurses or between doctors and nurses.

Notes

[1] A committee was appointed within the Ministry for Social Affairs in 1971 to help health and medical care authorities improve their planning and to make it easier to compare different health care areas and regions. The main job of this committee is to draw up a proposal for an organised system of hospital planning.

The planning system is intended to comprise three levels, with planning perspectives of thirty, fifteen, and five years. The first is an outline of nationwide development and expansion covering a thirty-year period; in turn, the county council's programmes will be based on this outline. The second covers fifteen years, and gives an aggregate plan for all the activities of the county councils, and a long-term budget. Goals, orientation, requirements, and resource forecasts for the different activities of the county councils are indicated in this overall plan. The third level covers five years and constitutes a plan for financing and operations. This level coincides with the county council's five-year budget.

217

This planning system is an extension of the continual forecasting programme of planning initiated by the Ministry for Social Affairs in 1967. Each year the county authorities submit to the Ministry their plans for the coming five-year period. These plans have included estimates of capacity and the number of visits in outpatient care, and the number of doctors and other medical staff needed, etc. Information on the need to educate medical staff, and cost estimates have also been covered by these plans.

[2] Patient groups have recently (1970-1972) begun to be more active. However, they have seldom questioned or influenced the hospital's strategic planning. Their main interest lies in matters related to the attention given to the patient's attitudes, and the way he is handled at the hospital, i.e. the doctors' behaviour during rounds, the patient's chances of being informed about the contents of his medical record, etc.

[3] SOU (The Swedish Government Official Reports), no. 4, 1962, *Tasks and Education for some Categories of Medical Personnel.* This official report was headed by G.F. Thapper, who was Speaker of the Swedish Parliament at the time. The report proposed a reallocation of tasks whereby some of the nurses' activities would be transferred to other personnel categories such as assistant nurses and ward clerks. This measure was aimed at alleviating the shortage of nurses. (It should be pointed out that there is no longer a shortage of nurses, except in certain specialised positions.)

[4] See note 3.

[5] The establishment of special clinics for the care of alcoholics was proposed in 1968 in SOU, no. 55, 1968, *Be Cured or Pay a Fine?.* This meant that care in these clinics would replace traditional police action by which intoxicated persons were taken into custody.

[6] Later, however, this proposal was rejected by the county council wages board.

[7] See note 8 to chapter 4.

[8] Data on the approximate number of persons involved were lacking in some instances. This reflects the fact that the persons proposing the various measures did not take the extent of these check-ups into account.

218

7 Administration of the Hospital's Production

The analysis of the administration of the hospital begun in the preceding chapter will now be extended to include the administration of production, i.e. management of the production system. We continue, first, by describing our hypotheses as to the demands which production and participant factors exert on the management and control of production. Then, under the assumption that these demands are met, we examine the administrative situation in the hospital itself.

At a very early stage in our study of the hospital, we noted that decisions made on medical matters by doctors and nurses were the most important element in the administration of the hospital. This decision making is necessary to satisfy the needs of the patients, and direct the utilisation of resources (internal and external efficiency; see chapter 2). The hospital's distinctive situation with respect to its production also places heavy demands on this decision making. In this chapter, when we describe and evaluate the decision making aimed at controlling the hospital's production—and this is mainly comprised of medical decision making—we deliberately use concepts unfamiliar to medical personnel. We will be talking about planning, processing, follow-up, control, etc. Systematic use of industrial concepts enables us to apply results from our own experience and research in different organisations. To help the reader, however, we shall begin with a more traditional description of the doctors' and nurses' work so as to illustrate the meaning of the concepts which will be used.

Medical decision making

The doctor traditionally describes his work in several phases: case history, diagnosis, therapy, and discharge. The approach we used in this study makes it more natural for us to distinguish only between decision making and treatment of patients. We thus classify the following as treatment: physical examination, laboratory tests, therapeutic and/or treatment measures, medication, surgery, and other measures involving direct contacts between the patient and hospital staff. However, these classifications

219

are not clear-cut. In any case, it is important to understand that since decision making and treatment of patients are processes which often take place simultaneously, it is difficult to break them down into definite stages. Attempts to make more realistic descriptions quickly lead to subdivisions into considerably more phases than those mentioned above. This is illustrated in Table 7.1, which describes the work of the doctors, and was compiled with the help of the department chiefs at General Hospital.[1]

However, the doctor is not the only person involved in medical decision making. The nurse and medical secretary act as assistants and are often responsible for the processing of important information and decision. The medical secretary is often the first person the patient comes in contact with, and on the basis of general instructions from the doctor, decides when a patient will be examined. The charge nurse makes many important decisions in conjunction with measures decided by the doctor.

There is a close connection between the decision making of nurses and doctors. One of the nurse's most demanding tasks—for example, in a medical department where many tests have to be performed—is to determine a suitable sequence for different diagnostic tests. A nurse gave the following example of how important it is to coordinate these kinds of decisions with those of the doctor:

> A patient had the following symptoms: diarrhoea, heart palpitation, and nausea. There were at least three possible explanations. The symptoms could be the result of the cardiac medication which the patient had been given. They could also be due to thyrotoxicosis or to malfunctioning of the gall bladder. The doctor ordered an X-ray of the gall bladder. The nurse suggested that they postpone the X-ray and perform a metabolism test first, to check the patient's thyroid. The doctor ordered both measures. The results showed that the metabolism test was abnormally high, while the gall bladder X-ray was negative. Unfortunately, the X-ray also made it impossible to administer any more metabolism tests for a whole year.[2]

We have used these examples to motivate our introductory statement that *medical decision making and the information processing related to it constitute the most important part of the administration of the hospital.*

The administration of production—our approach

If we define administration as information processing, and the administration of production as information processing aimed at managing the

220

TABLE 7.1

A doctor's description of the decisions and steps he goes through in treating a patient.

1	Basic patient data (national insurance papers, referral forms, previous records, X-rays, temperature chart, etc.)
2	Establishment of personal contact with the patient
3	Questions to the patient about the history of his illness
4	Physical examination
5	'Rough notes'
6	Notes (or impressions from memory) sorted
7	Records written (or dictated)
8	Preliminary diagnosis
9	Decision to supplementary diagnostic examinations and tests
10	Preliminary therapeutic decision
11	Notes on 8, 9, and 10 (in the medical record and on the temperature chart)
12	Entry into record of additional diagnostic results (tests)
13	Registration of the daily medical course of events (daily notes)
14	Reconsideration of preliminary diagnosis (possibly several times)
15	Reconsideration of preliminary therapy (possibly several times)
16	Evaluation prior to discharge
17	Instructions to the patient (and sometimes to relatives)
18	Information to the national insurance authorities and other institutions (medical, retirement, legal; health certificates, application for state subsidy for medical devices, etc.)
19	Information to referring physician or others who will take charge of the patient
20	Discharge summary (may be the same as step 19)
21	Registration of the diagnosis and preparation of the record
22	Medical record is filed

hospital's production, then it is obvious that both the doctors' and nurses' medical decision making can be regarded primarily as administration of production. In organisations which have a wide range of products and no possibilities for mass production—such as the hospital—some of the most important tasks related to management of production are:

1 to plan the extent of total production and distribute available resources between different production units (rough planning);

221

2 to determine what is required to attain the desired result with respect to each product (part of production processing);

3 to plan the sequence, time, and place for the execution of the different measures required for each individual product (detailed planning); and

4 to supervise the execution of decisions made (follow-up).

Various kinds of problems often arise in connection with these production administrative tasks. One of the most common problems is related to setting priorities and resolving the conflicts which result. Our study of the hospital's production had already convinced us that these different tasks had—or ought to have—their counterparts within the hospital. That which we term 'rough planning' should correspond most closely to planning for admission and to the admission process itself. Production processing is equivalent to decisions on treatment. Detailed planning and follow-up also have their counterparts in the work performed by doctors, nurses, and even medical secretaries.

Our approach is illustrated in the form of a flowchart which represents the administration of a goitre patient's treatment (Fig. 7.1). The key position of medical decision making in managing work in a hospital is clearly recognised. The flowchart also shows, however, that each decision made by a doctor is immediately followed by more or less complicated planning problems related to carrying out the decision. The patient has to be put on a waiting list, instructions have to be transferred in different directions, the patient has to be consulted, transport has to be arranged, and the execution of the various decisions has to be supervised. These administrative tasks are often delegated to a nurse or a secretary.

The hospital's production planning

Expectations

The hospital's uneven workload, and the limited interchangeability of the components, requires administrative flexibility. Forecasts of expected workload and production are important measures in this context. These can be used to plan admissions, inform patients and personnel, reallocate resources, etc. However, we formulated these expectations in very general terms. For example, we expected there to be summary forecasts for the hospital as a whole, and more detailed forecasts for the various clinical departments. Since production had such low predictability the drawing up

222

of long-term forecasts was made even more difficult. We expected less-detailed forecasts in connection with work on the annual budget, while the real basis for planning was short-term forecasts covering items such as the number of unoccupied beds during the coming week or month. We also expected to find long-term forecasts in connection with vacations and holidays.

Our expectations with respect to production planning were as follows:

(a) the smaller the number of emergencies, the more precise the planning of admissions;
(b) the wider the assortment and the greater the degree of internal specialisation (e.g. between different doctors), the more advantageous it becomes to plan the allocation of patients to different units within the clinical department;
(c) the greater the number of bottlenecks and unused capacity within a department (thus preventing rational use of resources), the greater the need for production planning for a more even workload;
(d) the simpler the products and the smaller the assortment, the more advantageous it becomes to admit several similar cases simultaneously.

Workload and production forecasts alone, however, cannot be expected to solve the hospital's planning problems. The variations in workload, and their low predictability, would in all likelihood still create disturbances in any planning system devised. But we were curious as to whether innovations had been made at the hospital which were unknown in other types of organisations. We expected one of the most important tasks of the hospital management to involve counteracting the low predictability in the production process.

The hospital's wide range of products, including many which both the hospital management and the participants regarded as secondary, made us expect that planning and other measures would be applied in deliberate attempts to allocate available resources between different products. In fact, we thought that without such measures, certain tasks or products (small, interesting, profitable) would be allotted more resources than intended and that others (large, uninteresting, less profitable) would receive less resources than intended (Gresham's law). We thus believed that a great deal of the actual management process would have to take place within the clinical departments. This is why we expected that special measures would be taken to indoctrinate the department chiefs about the hospital's views on priority allocation of resources between different types of tasks or products.

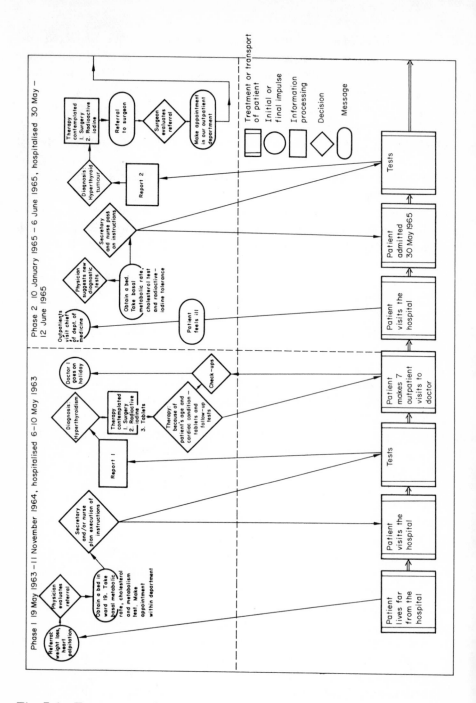

Fig. 7.1 Treatment of a goitre patient: decision detailed planning and follow-up.

224

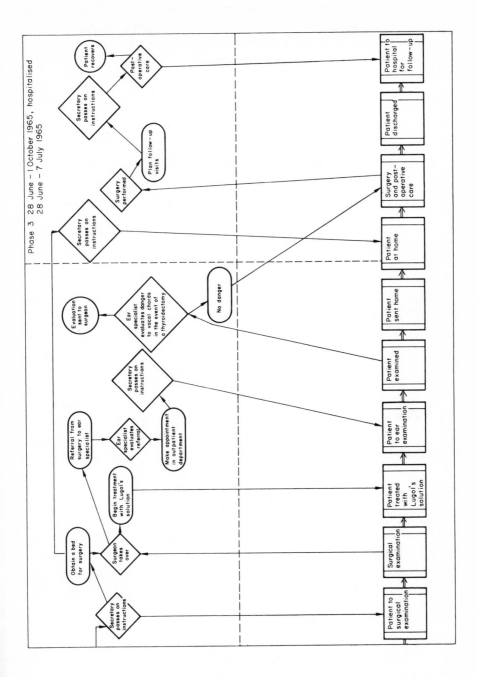

Phase 3 28 June – 1 October 1965, hospitalised
28 June – 7 July 1965

225

Finally, we expected that the hospital's high degree of self-sufficiency and its use of the market as an institution for cooperation and resolution of conflicts with suppliers would mean that material planning would be regarded as a simple administrative problem. We thought that one or several store-rooms and a simple purchasing routine would suffice.

Measurements

We ran into great difficulty trying to collect data about the hospital's and departments' methods of forecasting and planning for admissions and production. It seems clear that forecasting and planning are carried out in the clinical departments, generally by the department chief, although he is aided by the deputy department chief, junior physicians and nurses.

Simultaneous admission of several similar cases seldom occurs. It does take place, of course, during epidemics, but then it is not planned by the hospital. Treatment of hay fever and asthmatic school children as well as other allergies are to some extent handled in groups. Checks on reactions to X-ray therapy are sometimes carried out on a group of similar cases, for example in the form of group exercises (rehabilitation department) or group therapy (child psychiatry department). However, the department chiefs say that only a very small number of patients are treated in terms of some kind of 'mass production'. On the contrary, several of the department chiefs maintained that simultaneous admission of patients with similar illnesses was disadvantageous workwise and sometimes not indicated medically (for example owing to the increased danger of exposure).

The fact that the hospital is forced to close certain nursing units during vacations poses a special planning problem. The chief nurse is primarily responsible for this planning although the supervisory nurses and personnel department are also involved. We present a rather detailed description, in the chief nurse's own words, in order to illustrate how troublesome and time-consuming many planning problems become due to the shortage of personnel. The chief nurse's story should in fact be supplemented by the vivid descriptions of the misunderstandings which can arise made by the supervisory nurses, department chiefs, personnel assistants, charge nurses and others.

On the basis of previous lists, we start putting employees on different hours and schedules in order to handle the redistribution of working hours in the various clinical departments. A preliminary list of periods when the units will be closed is circulated so that information can be obtained from the departments and School of Nursing as to who is willing to substitute,

226

and when. The interplay between the prevailing shortage of teachers at the School of Nursing and students who are free to substitute is studied carefully. In this way the preliminary list of proposed periods when the units will be closed can be changed and specified in detail. After all departments have submitted changes, a preliminary closing schedule can be forwarded to the clinical departments and the School of Nursing. This usually takes place at the end of February.

Next, the doctors' holiday rota, and possibly other changes are submitted. This means that new personnel problems may arise due to a prevailing shortage of doctors. After changes have been entered, a proposed closing schedule is sent to all clinical departments, the vocational training school, the School of Nursing, the employment agency, department chiefs, and the board of trustees.

The board now deals with the closing schedule, and solves various predicaments which may have arisen, such as the closing of additional nursing units. After the board meeting, the closing schedule is sent to the press. The information is usually published in May and includes which units will be closed during the summer and precisely when. The closing schedule is then sent to the county Health and Medical Services Board.

Have any administrative innovations been made at the hospital which help counteract the effects of variations and unpredictability? We tried to evaluate these aspects by investigating reactions to various kinds of disturbances, and the measures taken to counteract them. Our expectations were partly met. The hospital uses a number of methods for counteracting disturbances in production. The most important is cyclical planning, which seems to have originated in hospitals long before it became widespread in industry.

Table 7.2 contains a survey of the cyclical course of events in in-patient care, and is based on a study made in the department of medicine. This table reveals that cyclical planning does not function without variations and disturbances. This should not be interpreted as criticism, however, since the most important purpose of cyclical planning is to show disturbances and other variations in a simple way. Overtime, overcapacity, changes in quality, and other measures at the hospital's disposal are included within the framework of the plan (see Table 7.3). Measures distinctive to the hospital primarily involve possibilities for varying the quality of products. There is a certain amount of leeway for adjusting to the workload—in the length of time allotted to care, the amount of time the doctor devotes to each patient, and the methods used. This does not have any counterpart in most industrial contexts.

Distribution of resources between different tasks, or groups of

227

TABLE 7.2

In-patient care routine (cyclical programme) at General Hospital

In-patient care routine (cyclical programme)	Frequency				Does the routine collide with other tasks		
	Daily	Weekly	Monthly	Other	Yes/No	If so, which?	Remarks
Rounds				Twice/day	Yes	Acute care, outpatient care	Afternoon work on the nursing unit is delayed
Menu	X				No		
Food, coffee, cleaning	X				No		
Patient appointments, telephone inquiries about patients	X				Yes	Afternoon tasks	
Laboratory tests (have to be given to laboratory at specific times)	X				Yes	Rounds and other morning tasks	
X-ray (request forms at the latest 7 p.m. the day before the X-rays are to be taken)	X				No		
X-ray (preparing patient for X-ray)	X				Yes	Rounds and other morning tasks	
Sterilisation of instruments	X				No		
Making beds				Three times/week	No		
Changing beds		X			No		
Baths (transport, bathing, and return of patients)		X			No		
Routine tests (every department has its own day for giving these to the laboratory,		X			No		
Inventory of instruments, dishes, and cutlery		X			No		
Supply lists		X			No		See above
Ordering supplies		X			No		See above
Spring cleaning				Yearly	No		In closed units during the summer vacation
Personnel budget proposals				Yearly	No		Adapted according to other

228

patients, is not regarded as a serious problem either by the county council or the hospital management. Six out of 12 interviewees, however, said that they suspected that outpatient care tended to take too many resources away from in-patients.[3]

The doctors were asked the same question and their attitudes were similar. When those who are critical of the way in which resources are allocated were asked to make their answers more specific, their replies varied greatly (Fig. 7.2). Attempts to find a variable which might explain the difference between doctors' opinions have been unsuccessful. The distribution within groups of department chiefs and junior doctors, older and younger doctors, doctors in departments with an emphasis on outpatient care, and those with limited outpatient care, is about the same as in the population as a whole.

About half the doctors and nurses think that the allocation of resources poses a problem for them personally and they usually criticise themselves for the mistakes they make in dividing their time between different tasks

TABLE 7.3

The hospital's adaption to disturbances and variations in workload

Disturbances	Ways of counteracting disturbances
Variations originating outside the hospital	
Increased patient flow in outpatient units.	Extra workload, with patients waiting in line, or unused capacity.
Need to examine outpatients more thoroughly.	Problems of coordination with other units. Strains on the service departments. Also affects nursing units.
Outpatient emergencies.	Either regular patients or emergencies have to wait.
Increased flow of patients needing in-patient care.	Waiting lists (number of beds is fixed).
Need to examine patients more closely and give them more therapy in the nursing units.	Number of personnel allocated according to the greatest possible workload. Stress and strain in the units, or unused capacity.
Increased patient flow during the night.	Extra workload for on-call doctors and nurses.

229

Table 7.3 (continued)

Patients arriving at the X-ray department during lunch hour.	Longer waiting time for patient.
Employee absenteeism.	Shortage of resources in units or out-patient departments, with possibly longer waiting times for patients.
Drug salesmen wanting to see the doctor immediately.	Underutilisation of other medical resources and longer waiting time for patients.

Variations originating within the hospital

Supplies in the various departments used up.	Shortages can arise. Store-room personnel may have to transport supplies; otherwise, there is poor use of resources or poor quality of care.
Differences in workload between units in the hospital.	Some resources not fully utilised, others show abnormal wear and tear.
Large number of cases that a doctor has to cover during X-ray rounds.	Redeployment of doctors, with the exception of the radiologist.
Variation in the time required for rounds in the department.	If a doctor, especially the department chief or his assistant, has surgery afterwards, longer waiting time may arise in operating rooms.
Variation in the time at which rounds begin.	Poor use of resources in the nursing unit.
Need to make laboratory tests late in the day.	Extra workload in the laboratory.
Heavy workload in the X-ray department.	Unused capacity or waiting lists. In-patients have to wait for X-rays. This, in turn, can mean that the patient remains on a nursing unit with no treatment or progress in his condition.
Lack of reliability in filing, and variations in the product from the secretarial pool.	Extra work for doctors, perhaps resulting in unsatisfactory records.

230

and patient groups. Figure 7.3 shows that our expectations were well realised as to the types of problem reported. Simple cases, 'irrelevant cases' (such as psychosomatic and social welfare cases), telephone and paperwork all intrude and take working time away from the most important tasks, such as in-patient care and special cases relevant to individual research.

Tables 7.2 and 7.3 and Figs. 7.2 and 7.3 do not, of course, indicate that half the doctors and nurses do not have the problems mentioned. Someone who replies 'No' to the question 'Do you usually criticise yourself for distributing your working time between different types of patients or tasks in a way you feel is unsuitable?' might be highly criticised by an observer for his use of working time. However, the answers do indicate how people evaluate their own situation.

Even though our expectations were met, i.e. Gresham's law can be regarded as a problem, both the county council and the hospital management have done little to change conditions which they did not think were desirable. A spokesman for the county council claimed that, at least in regard to certain department chiefs, it was impossible to interfere since the outpatient clinics were really the department chiefs' private offices. The best solution entails establishing new units devoted to outpatient care. In the long term, health centres and group practices will have to be expanded and constructed to lessen the workload in the hospital's outpatient departments.

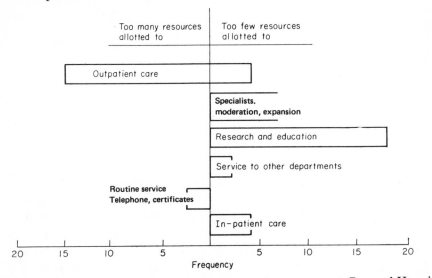

Fig. 7.2 Doctors' opinions as to allocation of resources at General Hospital.

231

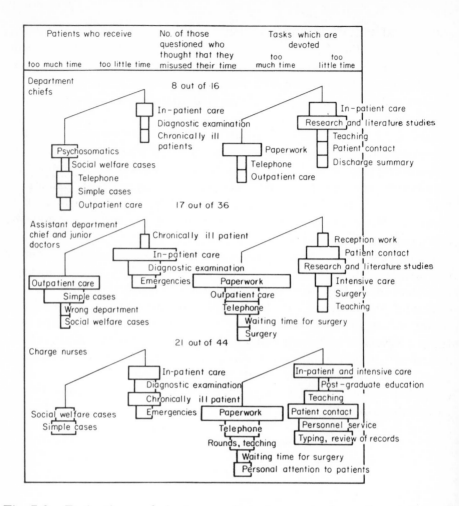

Fig. 7.3 Evaluations of doctors and nurses as to how they use, and misuse, their working time.

Cyclical planning (by which we mean scheduling of recurring activities, especially the weekly routine) is one way in which the use of time and the distribution of resources can be influenced within the clinical departments. Their distribution between in-patients and outpatients is affected, for example, by devoting certain days or hours each week to outpatient care.[4] Time and motion studies had not been used before at General Hospital to obtain more detailed knowledge on the use of resources for different types of tasks. Nor had there been any cost accounting on a product basis.

One special problem involves the arrangements required for the continued education of doctors and for research. There are many different opinions within the county council, the board of trustees, and among the department chiefs, with respect to these matters. The county council gave a 25,000 cr. grant to General Hospital for research. Slightly less than half the department chiefs said that they had made special arrangements to promote research and education—but if they did so, their efforts were usually very modest. Of course, rounds, X-ray rounds, staff meetings, and daily treatment are mentioned, though several doctors claim that leave of absence for research work is seldom granted, special study trips are not very common, and little or no equipment has been acquired for research purposes. One department chief who was highly interested in research said: 'Leave of absence for research is granted only as a rare exception. No special research appointments have been made. When the members of the medical staff make their daily rounds, they meet and discuss recent scientific and medical advances. A junior doctor is usually asked to talk on a particular topic and give a resumé of an article or paper.'

Another department chief, who was highly interested in the education of his subordinates, stated: 'Leave of absence is granted for research. When courses are held, permission is requested for suitable employees to participate. At least four such courses have been attended by employees from my department during the past year.'

But this is an exception. Sixty per cent of the junior doctors are dissatisfied with the arrangements made for research and post-graduate training by the clinical departments. They also made new proposals, such as:

Allotting time daily to further education by keeping abreast of current literature. Specialty meetings once a week for discussions of theoretical principles (there is not enough time for this at present).

Intensive post-graduate training as in the American training system, with

a   Postgraduate lectures
b   Grand rounds
c   Bedside instruction
d   Instruction at the operating table
e   More conferences

More opportunities for conferences among doctors. More reviews of journals, and preferably, some kind of research and/or special study programme.

233

I would like the doctors in each department to devote an hour or two each week to discussing cases, diagnostic methods, and so on.

We studied the planning for supplies by interviewing the employees responsible for these matters at General Hospital. It turned out that our expectations were met to a large extent. Articles in regular use are stored centrally at the hospital, at the place where they are used, or both. Forecasts of when orders should be placed, and of quantities to be bought, are determined on the basis of the previous year's consumption. Store-room accounts were transferred to automatic data processing in October 1965, which means that the purchasing department now receives information more rapidly with regard to the necessity of placing new orders. Articles which are not kept in stock are bought on request by a department as the need arises, and after checking and approval by the chief nurse.

Food, fuel oil, and certain other items are bought centrally by the county council's purchasing department. Furniture and equipment for the clinical departments are bought in accordance with special inventory surveys. Laundry is delivered in two ways, either on order to the various units, or through automatic replacements from the central laundry to local supply-rooms.

Central purchasing is relatively new, and the purchasing department is not yet fully recognised as a necessary service. A charge nurse made the following comments (some doctors made similar statements):

It always takes such a long time to get new articles nowadays. First you have to ask for bids, and after that it takes at least six months before you receive anything. You 'hand in your requisition in triplicate, etc.' instead of simply going to a firm, looking at an item, and buying it as we used to do. It's understandable that there has to be some kind of control of purchases from a budgeting point of view, but the way things are now, it's very inconvenient. If you call the purchasing department and ask for something, they don't even know what it's used for.

However, on the basis of this and other similar complaints, it is impossible to conclude how well central purchasing really functions. In any case, its status seems to be low—this indirectly confirms our expectations with regard to material planning.

234

The hospital's production planning (treatment procedures)

Expectations

One of the most important characteristics of the hospital's situation is what was referred to in chapter 5 as a 'wide product assortment'. The discussion in chapter 5 resulted in the observation that, even if patients can be classified according to certain types of illnesses, this is merely an ex post construction. When a patient first comes in contact with the hospital, the type of illness he suffers from is generally not clear. Therefore, every patient has to be regarded as an individual in terms of his diagnosis. This situation guided most of our expectations about the hospital's treatment procedure.

We more or less expected the wide assortment to lead to individual treatment procedures. We assumed that low predictability would make it difficult, or uneconomic, to decide—before treatment was begun—on all the procedures which would be applied up to the time when the patient was discharged. However, since the costs of different treatment procedures have to be considered, we expected that efforts would sometimes be made to reduce them, e.g. through standard procedures. Demands for individual treatment and standard procedures necessitate a compromise.

The wide assortment implies that the doctor has to be able to evaluate a large number of alternatives. This means that information about available alternatives and their consequences has to be easily accessible. Thus, we expected doctors to have ready access to information about possible therapeutic measures through reference books and similar works. To the extent that alternatives which were medically equivalent were available, we expected that the costs of these alternatives would be regarded as rather unimportant, and that the doctors would not be very well informed about the costs of treatment alternatives.

Low predictability leads to successive decisions on treatment procedures. The patient's medical history and previous treatment are important bases for new decisions. Therefore, we expected the filing system and communication aids to be highly important. We also expected to find use of automatic data processing for treatment procedures—or that its introduction would be contemplated.

Another result of the wide assortment is that the work involved in treatment procedures requires great and varied efforts which increase in direct proportion to the complexity of the product. The large number of doctors required by the hospital to handle the innumerable treatment procedures are dispersed in many independent clinical departments. This

235

tends to eliminate the possibility of central coordination or control of individual cases. Follow-up supervision is also troublesome because of the difficulty inherent in measuring quality. Therefore, we expected the hospital management to devote a great deal of attention to indoctrinating common guidelines and quality norms for treatment procedures. For example, we expected to find written guidelines, internal education, etc. We also anticipated that the guidelines set up for medical decision making would be closely regulated as part of the personnel system, to include principles for wages, recruitment, and promotions. On the basis of what was said earlier about the hospital's distinctive participant relations, we did not expect indoctrination about cost consciousness to be highly developed.

Finally, we expected the wide assortment and the introduction of new techniques to make it difficult to maintain the planners'—especially that of the doctors'—medical knowledge and problem-solving ability. On the basis of conditions in other organisations with a heavy emphasis on administrative problem solving, we expected to find special measures within the hospital which are aimed at improving, maintaining, and utilising the physicians' capacity and ability as problem solvers. Our most important expectations in this context were as follows:

1   A great deal of resources would be reserved for post-graduate studies for physicians.
2   To the extent that the shortage of staff makes it necessary to work with inexperienced or partly trained personnel, special training programmes would be made available. Substitutes and newly hired personnel would be given a special induction.
3   There would be internal specialisation among doctors so that each would be responsible for certain groups of patients, the less qualified being responsible for simple cases, the more experienced doctors responsible for difficult cases.
4   The most highly qualified doctors would be completely exempt from routine tasks.
5   There would be extensive medical conferences and consultation.

Measurements

We had a great deal of difficulty in studying treatment procedures, especially in diagnostic work; this is partly because they took us into purely medical matters. Therefore, we had to be satisfied with general observa-

236

tions and information gathered through interviews, mainly with the doctors and nurses. This is regrettable, because the study of treatment procedures seems to constitute one of the most important factors in evaluating the administration of the hospital.

A great deal of the production within the hospital is carried out according to standard procedures. In the nursing units, this applies to everything linked with the hospital's 'hotel function', i.e. serving meals, washing dishes, cleaning, etc. Figure 7.4 shows that the 'hotel function' constitutes a large part of the total work of the nursing units. Standard procedures have been established to regulate these tasks. The times when these tasks should be carried out, and the relevant division of labour, are also planned in relation to the hospital's daily routine (Table 7.4). However, standard procedures extend far beyond the hospital's hotel function. We were very impressed by how advanced the hospital was in training its employees to carry out these standard procedures, some being outlined for nurses in a procedure handbook. Table 7.5 shows the chapter headings in this handbook. Figure 7.5 is an example of one of the standard procedures included in the handbook, which is intended for student nurses and nurses who have been away from nursing for some years.

The procedures for doctors are more numerous and specialised than for nurses. But since General Hospital is not a teaching hospital, and since there are only a few doctors in each clinical department, there does not seem to be much need to compile procedures in handbooks (reference books are discussed below.)

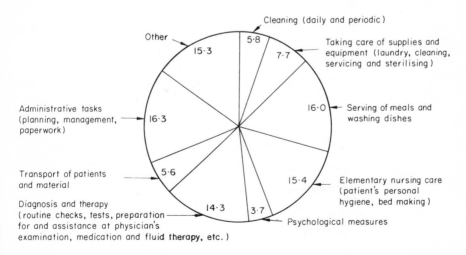

Fig. 7.4 The distribution of working time among various types of tasks in a surgical nursing unit at General Hospital.

237

Standard procedures enable the person in charge of a particular treatment to give rather brief and general instructions, at least for some kinds of treatment and care. The doctor's job is mainly to select from the procedures he and his colleagues have learned. Thus, his instructions to the nurse may often be very brief: 'Prepare for surgery', 'Give an intravenous', 'Do a TB test'.

Treatment procedures can also be programmed to some extent. Medical histories and social welfare reports for certain categories of patients are standardised and are usually made by younger members of staff or helpers, such as social workers. Certain tests are performed routinely on all patients in most clinical departments. Figure 7.6 is an example of the

TABLE 7.4

The routine at General Hospital includes this 'daily schedule'.

1 Nursing staff begin at 7 a.m., possibly 7.30 or later, and finish at 9 p.m., possibly 9.30 or earlier, in accordance with the working schedule.

2 Patients are awakened by night staff at 6 a.m. Lights are turned off by the day staff at 9 p.m.

3 Mealtimes for patients: breakfast 8.15 a.m., lunch 12 noon, dinner 4.30 p.m., snacks 7 to 8 p.m., for employees: breakfast 7 to 9 a.m., lunch 11 a.m. to 1 p.m., dinner 4 to 5 p.m.

4 Rounds are made in the morning between 8 and 10 a.m., and in the afternoon from 3 to 3.30 p.m.

5 Rest hour, 1 to 2 p.m.

6 Visiting hours Wednesday, Saturday, and Sunday 2 to 3 p.m., Tuesday and Thursday 6.30 to 7 p.m.

7 Telephone inquiries about patients 1 to 3 p.m.

8 Special office hours for admissions personnel, wages department, store-room, pharmacy, library, maintenance, baths, and outpatient departments.

9 Night clinic opens at 8 p.m.

way in which diagnostic work is standardised in the outpatient unit of the department of medicine.

Standard treatment procedures are seldom written down. They are passed on verbally when new employees are taught 'how we do things in this clinical department'. Since staff turnover is lower for doctors than nurses, the nurses become agents of tradition. The charge nurses sometimes maintained that one of their jobs was to tell 'the young junior doctors that the department chief would be very happy if this and that test were performed before he came'.

We have used these examples to illustrate how a compromise takes place between individual and standard treatment. Thus, we were surprised

TABLE 7.5

The procedure handbook contains some of the standard procedures
a nurse has to perform

1 Intravenous infusion
2 Subcutaneous infusion
3 Catheterisation and bladder irrigation of female patients
4 Catheterisation and bladder irrigation of male patients
5 Giving enemas
6 Temperature taking
7 Ewald's test breakfast (simplified method)
8 Fractional examination of gastric juices with caffeine solution and, if necessary, injection of histamines
9 Fractional examination of gastric juices with histamines
10 Care of patient after death
11 Shaving
12 Routine tests in the most common medical illnesses
13 Routine tests in the most common surgical illnesses
14 Serving meals
15 Giving oxygen
16 Giving additional oxygen in new nursing units
17 Instructions for cooperation with X-ray department
18 Recording temperature curve
19 Decontamination
20 Bathing methods
21 Taking samples from contagious patients

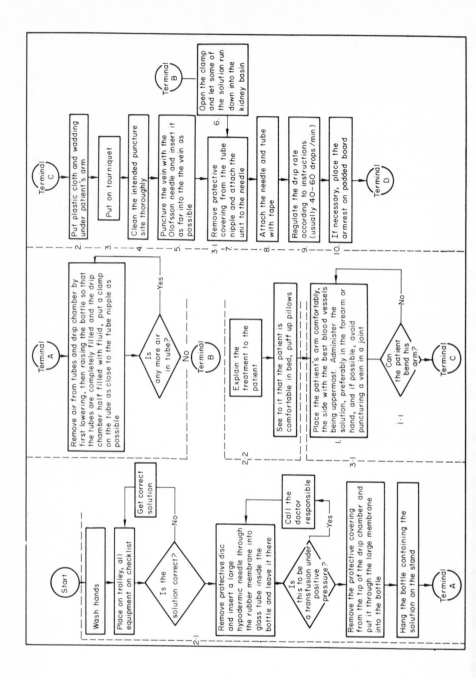

240

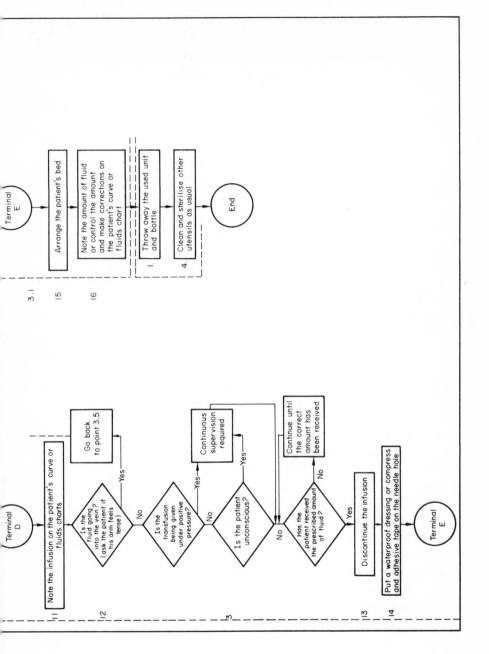

Fig. 7.5 Intravenous infusion procedure as in the procedure handbook at General Hospital.

that neither the department chiefs nor the chief nurse seemed aware of the need for compromise. In any case, experiments or studies are seldom made in these matters. One possible explanation is that new methods for treatment procedures are regarded as medical innovations that the doctors do not believe they can introduce on their own. Instead, they depend on developments taking place in teaching hospitals, research institutes, etc. This explanation was suggested by several interviewees. Another possible explanation, arrived at on the basis of some profitability analyses which we made with respect to increased and decreased standardisation of treatment procedures, is that the cost curve is rather flat, i.e. that little is to be earned from the economic standpoint by increasing or decreasing the number of routine tests, for example.

A review of standard procedures, such as routine tests, is generally made only when new department chiefs (or assistant department chiefs) begin work at the hospital. Then everything is accomplished very simply. One department chief said: 'When I arrived, I simply posted a list of the tests that were standard.'

All the important aspects of our expectations about the hospital's information system were realised. A great deal of attention was given to the writing of medical records. Every clinical department had its own files, and even if some of the doctors were far from satisfied with the way in which their records were kept and functioned, we as outsiders could not but be impressed by the strict order which was maintained.

There were no plans to use computers for medical purposes—but advances in this area were being watched carefully. The doctor in charge of the laboratories at General Hospital has been appointed by the county council as adviser to a study dealing with the future acquisition of computers.

The most important telecommunication aids at the hospital are the telephone and an intercom system. There was at least one secretary in each clinical department, and most of the doctors use dictaphones. Medical secretaries constitute a problem in several departments, mainly because there are too few of them.

The doctors have access to high-quality reference books containing information as to the medical consequences of different alternatives of action. The 'Synonym Handbook' contains a list of pharmaceuticals, including comparisons of equivalent or 'synonomous' drugs. 'Current Therapy' is a reference series full of information about instructions for diagnosis and treatment. There are two copies of this series at the hospital, but they are not used by more than a few doctors. New junior doctors are better acquainted with their textbooks, and often consult them first

242

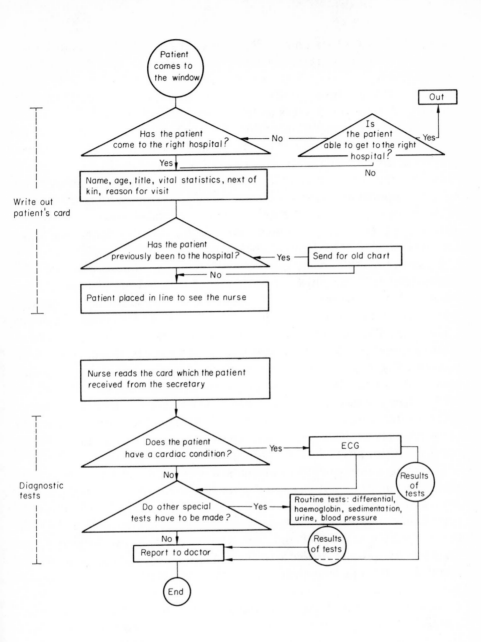

Fig. 7.6 Standard procedure for secretaries and nurses in outpatient departments at General Hospital.

243

before turning to other sources. When doctors require additional information, they frequently try to get hints from their colleagues during discussions at lunch.

Cost estimates for a specific treatment procedure are never made in advance. Most of the doctors seem to think that these kinds of deliberations conflict with professional ethics. In informal interviews, however, we observed that rough economic evaluations do provide a basis for allocating priority of use for certain scarce resources at the hospital. These 'economic' considerations cover a patient's age, his profession, chances of returning to his job, opportunities for re-education, etc. Cost accounting which provides ex post information about different types of costs, or costs for different patients, is performed only in the so-called operating costs accounts which will be described below.

We attempted to measure the doctors' knowledge of costs more specifically. About half the physicians at General Hospital answered ten questions, and a 'knowledge of costs index' which we constructed revealed that it would be possible to reduce costs by 30 per cent in the situations under study if all doctors had complete knowledge about costs. However, these inquiries provided an insight into the difficulties of simulating situations leading to comparable alternatives of action. If choices between equivalent drugs with different prices are disregarded, then doctors are seldom faced with decision situations in which the medical consequences of two alternatives are completely comparable.[5] Thus, possible lack of knowledge about costs cannot be expected to be of much importance in terms of the hospital's total costs.

Our expectation that there would be a need to indoctrinate the doctors about certain common goals and policies was not met. It seemed only natural that the hospital management would not be involved in this task, particularly because of what was said in the preceding chapter, i.e. that the hospital management did not devote much effort to policy formulation. It was also difficult to find any conscious effort by doctors to establish goals and guidelines. There were few written instructions (see Table 7.6).

Most of the junior doctors and charge nurses admitted that their department chiefs seldom, or never, discussed matters of principle with them. One important exception, however, concerned methods of diagnosis and treatment (see Table 7.7).

Our lack of medical knowledge made it difficult for us to measure—or even evaluate—the consequences of so little attention being paid to formulating common policies. But we did find that many younger doctors were highly critical of the fact that so little time was devoted to discussing

244

matters of principle. On several occasions we asked groups of doctors about their obligations with respect to rounds. This turned out to be an excellent question for stimulating a discussion; the doctors were highly uncertain about activities which we assumed to be exceedingly important.

Very often the doctors did not know the correct regulations and their opinions differed from the 'rules currently in effect'. One department chief claimed that he had solved the problem of rounds in the afternoons by simply cancelling them. He said that he was not aware that there were any regulations about rounds. Another doctor who made rounds several times a day, thought that the only existing regulation was that the doctor should inform himself of the patients' condition every day. A third doctor thought that there was a rule that rounds should be made twice a day at times stipulated in the

TABLE 7.6

The frequency of written instructions at General Hospital

Question to department chiefs:
To what extent have written instructions been formulated *in your* clinical department for any of the following tasks?

		No. of department chiefs who have formulated instructions	No. of department chiefs who intend to have instructions formulated
a	Behaviour of employees towards patients		1
b	Behaviour of employees towards relatives of patients		1
c	Behaviour of different groups of employees towards each other		1
d	Activity of junior doctors in outpatient care	2	1
e	Research within the department	2	1
f	Education of junior doctors and student nurses	2	1
g	Criteria for admission		1
h	Diagnostic methods	5	
i	Treatment methods	4	
j	Records	6	1
k	Donation of blood	1	
l	Dispensing of drugs	1	

245

daily schedule, while a fourth thought this to be completely wrong. He assumed that the daily schedule was aimed at protecting the nurses, i.e. rounds were not permitted at hours other than those stipulated.

Matters of medical policy were seldom discussed by the department chiefs' association. As was shown in the preceding chapter, basic norms and values are not created and maintained by the doctors at the hospital, but rather by an international and national professional corps.

The National Board of Health and Welfare could possibly be regarded as an authority with the power to set up norms, though most of the doctors are inclined to perceive this board as an interpreter of the norms and values of the medical corps. We tried in two—equally unsatisfactory—ways to find out about some of the norms and values which guide the doctor as a decision maker. By asking 'How can we evaluate whether your department is well organised?' we tried to find where the physician seeks his points of reference.[6]

Are the attitudes of colleagues, patients, or employees the most important? Table 7.8 reveals more market- and employee-oriented answers than we had expected. This table is based on a questionnaire, though supplementary interviews confirmed that more department chiefs than we

TABLE 7.7

Discussion of matters of policy and principle at General Hospital.

Question to junior doctors: Has your department chief ever discussed with you principles for . . .	Never	Once or twice	Regularly
Behaviour of employees towards patients	18	14	2
Behaviour of employees towards relatives	24	10	–
Behaviour of different groups of employees towards each other	18	15	1
Junior doctors' activities in outpatient care	8	17	10
Research within the department	17	13	2
Education of junior doctors or student nurses	14	16	5
Criteria for admission	14	11	9
Diagnostic methods	3	12	20
Treatment methods	3	11	21
Principles for treating emergencies	10	11	13
Medical records	18	12	4
Division of work in the department	10	20	5
Working time and performance norms for junior doctors	14	13	6

had thought wanted to seek their evaluations outside the medical profession. A typical answer is as follows:

> Well, that's a difficult question. Of course, this kind of evaluation had to be made from the point of view of both employees and patients. I'd have to go around and ask the employees. And as for the patients, I guess I'd have to do the same and ask them whether they were feeling better and what opinions they had about the care they have received.

However, professional orientation is observed in answers of the following type:

> A good department is one where you can employ capable junior doctors. This presupposes that the department chief is proficient, and willing to educate his colleagues.
> The first prerequisite of a well-organised department is that its patients are satisfied. But this is not enough—the treatment administered also has to be medically correct.

Question to charge nurses: Has your department chief ever discussed with you principles for . . .	Never	Once or twice	Regularly
Behaviour of employees towards patients	26	14	–
Behaviour of employees towards relatives	29	9	–
Behaviour of different groups of employees towards each other	27	11	1
Methods of care and treatment	7	13	20
Educational matters (e.g. of student nurses)	18	15	3
Hygiene in the department	17	18	5
Division of work in the department	22	16	1
Rationalisation	22	10	6
Drug consumption	20	14	5

A comparison of the doctors' and nurses' answers, however, shows that the nurses are more market- or patient-oriented than are the doctors (see Table 7.8).

As well as this simple measurement, we made systematic observations to reach conclusions about the norms and values which guide the doctors. The following are some excerpts from our pilot study, which, after having completed the study as a whole, we still believe are representative.

One of the notions sometimes expressed in the general debate is that hospital employees are more conservative and more opposed to change than are other employees, particularly those in industrial firms. The doctors at General Hospital have often accused the nurses of this attitude, and the administrative staff sometimes made the same complaint against both nurses and doctors. The younger doctors also felt the same way about the older doctors. But we did not get the impression that these observations are warranted. Changes are usually accepted quite willingly in the field of medicine. We also found more examples of nurses actively involved in bringing about changes than the contrary. Obviously, however, employees familiar with a certain 'repertoire' are not willing to give it up without good reason. Thus, we find it easy to agree with the criticism that nurses sometimes reacted against 'change for its own sake' and against the lack of information distributed in conjunction with impending changes.

TABLE 7.8

What should an evaluation of whether a department is well-organised be based on?

What are the most important conditions to take into account in evaluating whether a department is well organised?		Professional staff	Satisfied personnel	Satisfied patients	Good organisation	No answer
		(%)	(%)	(%)	(%)	(%)
Department chiefs	16 respondents	50	25	6	13	6
Charge nurses	63 respondents	10	37	21	14	19
Other supervisors	28 respondents	25	32	7	21	14

248

One important norm for which the doctors differ greatly from heads of industrial firms is that of being on time. Punctuality at the hospital is far from being as self-evident as it is in an industrial firm. Almost without exception, we found that doctors and nurses are extremely lenient in accepting that they and others, ourselves included, did not succeed in adhering to time estimates and appointed times. This applies to relations between patients and colleagues alike. We often felt uncomfortable knowing that patients were sitting in the waiting-room. But the doctors were completely unmoved. In our turn, we often had to sit and wait for the doctor even though we had an appointment.

Work is fun. Work is a duty. One should work until all tasks have been completed. In any case, these norms apply to all work that has to do with acutely ill patients and emergencies. On the other hand, we also found examples of doctors believing that they had a right to 'educate' patients who made demands which they did not consider legitimate (such as appearing at the night clinic without suffering from acute symptoms). But this is an exception. Most patients who come to the hospital require care. The employees are aware of this. For instance, it is unusual for service units—which are remote from the patient—to refuse to participate owing to their workload, over-time, etc.

The salary system of department heads and junior doctors is a stimulus to hard work and gives priority to outpatient rather than in-patient care.[7] The doctors are divided into two 'income blocs' in this respect. One group has significant, and the other insignificant, income from outpatient care. Many charge nurses are highly critical of outpatient care and the doctors' involvement in it. A few depart-ment chiefs are generally regarded (even among the doctors) as spending too much time in outpatient care and instead, delegating almost all in-patient care and supervision of their departments to the assistant department chief and junior doctors. Young doctors have also confided that outpatients are sometimes treated in a manner aimed at ensuring the doctor as large an income as possible. It has been pointed out to us that the patients almost always have to wait, the nurses often have to wait—but never the doctors. Sometimes, patients are told to return for another visit which is not entirely necessary, but which gives the doctor an easily earned income. How-ever, we have a strong impression that these statements apply to

249

isolated exceptions. There is no justification for alluding to general misuse—except perhaps with respect to doctors' punctuality. The most important reason for this seems to be peer group control. Doctors have strong values which rank the patient and care first, and condemn any physician who visibly violates this norm.

The doctors at General Hospital seem to evaluate patient care and clinical work more highly than research. Everyone was aware of the fact that research paid off in the physician's career. But colleagues still appreciated and respected a 'good clinician' more than a 're-searcher'. We found that some doctors were directly hostile towards research. 'It doesn't belong in a county hospital.'

The necessity of keeping costs down was not discussed to any great extent; or at least, it was seldom discussed between the department chiefs and employees in the clinical departments. Fifty per cent of department chiefs admitted this openly, and we have reason to suspect that the eight who said that they sometimes discuss costs with their employees tend to over-estimate their efforts in this area. In any case, there was very poor agree-ment between statements made by the employees and the department chiefs. This merely slight interest in reducing costs, however, does agree with our expectations. We said previously that this is not among the most important demands made on the hospital. Indoctrinating the staff with a demand for cost consciousness would simply be inappropriate to the given situation.

Naturally, it is an extremely difficult and delicate task to evaluate whether sufficient and suitable action is taken at General Hospital in regard to using and maintaining the doctors' medical knowledge and pro-blem-solving ability. Again, we were forced to rely on informal measure-ments, and had little access to data which were not already well known to anyone acquainted with a hospital. On the other hand, our method, which involves comparisons with other types of organisations, does imply that certain general observations might be of value. The most important are:

1 The junior doctor's career—which, in addition to the formal basic education, includes extensive practical training and rotation between different clinical departments and hospitals, sometimes circulating between county and university hospitals—is superior to a career in most other professions in terms of creating and maintaining professional know-ledge. For a long time, doctors seem to have had a system similar to that which the most advanced large firms are just now experimenting with for engineers and economists.

250

2   This systematic medical education diminishes, or comes to an end, when a doctor receives an appointment as a department chief. Further education for department chiefs consists mainly of courses and conventions arranged by different medical and scientific organisations. However, this depends entirely on the department chiefs own initiative. Several of those interviewed did not think that further education was appreciated by the county council or the hospital management. 'If you want to get away for a course they regard it as a disruption for one's colleagues.' 'We don't get any compensation or thanks for studying more.' 'Further education which is regarded as an expression of scientific interest is not especially popular in the county council.'[8]

3   However, if we accept the opinions of junior doctors, lack of up-to-date knowledge appears to pose few problems. We found that only a few junior doctors thought their knowledge superior to their chief's. We are fairly sure that different answers would have been given if young engineers or economists had been asked to compare their knowledge with that of their older colleagues. The lack of a problem in this sphere may, to some extent, be explained by the fact that department chiefs are usually appointed fairly late in life.[9]

4   In the junior doctors' opinion, locums are not given a satisfactory induction in most clinical departments.

5   The division into clinical departments itself implies internal specialisation among doctors. In addition, there is formal internal specialisation.

6   The doctors' salary system discourages a suitable division of work because compensation per hour in outpatient care is less in the more difficult cases. Another reason is that a fixed salary is paid for work in the in-patient units where the need for qualified medical care is greatest. A large group of junior doctors (44 per cent) thought that this results in an unsuitable division of work whereas most department chiefs (13 out of 15) do not believe that this presents a serious problem.

7   The most-qualified doctors are not wholly exempt from routine tasks. The doctors themselves think that 5 to 25 per cent of the tasks they now perform could be transferred to other, less-qualified personnel.

8   Almost half the department chiefs are not completely satisfied with the present system for specialist consultations between the doctors at the hospital. They complain about having to wait for consultations, and also think that written consultations do not provide enough personal contact. Two department chiefs also said they regretted that time does not allow them to make satisfactory contributions to consultations. Another problem arises during the summer when most doctors are away and locums

251

take over. This means that patients are referred to different specialists to a much greater extent than usual.

9 The doctors are dissatisfied with the scope of their medical conferences and consultations. They suggested many new types of medical conferences which are non-existent today. Table 7.9 shows the medical conferences which now take place. Figure 7.7 indicates wishes expressed by the physicians with regard to conferences.

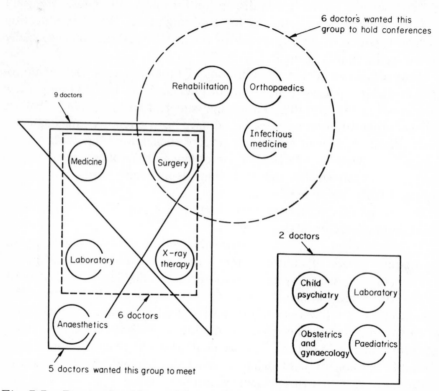

Fig. 7.7 Doctors' wishes with regard to medical conferences at General Hospital.

Patient planning at the hospital

Expectations

The wide assortment, heavy workload, and varying demands on delivery time (i.e. a large proportion of emergencies) and the high labour costs of products (resulting from the high service content) all contribute to making

TABLE 7.9

Medical conferences at General Hospital during 1965 with participants from more than one department (DC = Department chief)

Subject	Participants	Frequency	Approx. length
1. Polio unit	DC infectious medicine + DC orthopaedics	1/month	8 hours
2. Selected cases	DC infectious medicine + DC chest	1 to 2/month	
3. CP paediatric cases	DC paediatrics + CP personnel	1/week	2 hours
4. Orthopaedics conference	Physician from rehabilitation + DC orthopaedics	1/week .	$\frac{1}{2}$ to $\frac{3}{4}$ hour
5. Vocational training conference	Physicians from rehabilitation and psychiatry + psychologist + occupational therapist + employee from vocational training centre + possibly other specialists	1 to 2/week	$1\frac{1}{2}$ hour
6. Abortion conference	Physicians from psychiatry and gynaecology	1/week	1 hour
7. Chemistry lab. rounds	Department of medicine + chemistry lab.	2/week	$\frac{1}{4}$ hour
8. Isotope lab. rounds	X-ray therapy + surgeon + physician from department of medicine	1 to 2/week	$\frac{1}{4}$ hour
9. X-ray rounds	X-ray physician + physicians from surgery, medicine, orthopaedics, ear, nose and throat, chest, paediatrics, long-term care, infectious medicine	Daily (pulmonary and ear: 1/week	$\frac{1}{4}$ to $\frac{1}{2}$ hour
10. Rounds in intensive care unit	DC anaesthesties + long-term care + physicians from surgery and medicine	Daily	10 minutes
11. Staff meetings	All physicians at the hospital and physicians in the area are invited	1/week	1 to $1\frac{1}{2}$ hour

253

detailed planning—primarily the determination of when and where a patient should be treated—an important task. The more complicated a case, and the more dependent a clinical department is on other departments and service units (i.e. the lower the degree of autonomy), the more time-consuming detailed planning becomes and the greater the need for follow-up activities. Thus, wide differences between these activities in the clinical departments can be expected. We expected these differences to mean that special resources would be allotted to detailed planning and follow-up activities in the departments with the least autonomy and the highest degree of complexity.

Cooperation between employees is complicated and changeable due to the wide assortment of relatively complex products and low predictibility. With some exaggeration, it can be said that everyone in the hospital is dependent on immediate help from anyone at almost any time. In the more autonomous clinical departments, this interdependency exists primarily within departments themselves, whereas the less autonomous departments are more dependent on the service units. The difficulty of establishing a standardised flow of products and simple forms of cooperation requires an informal and complicated authority structure. Thus, we did not expect the hospital to have job descriptions, an outline of the chain of command, a description of the decision-making process, and other formal instructions as to 'who may give orders to whom'.

Measurements

It turned out to be difficult for us to use the methods available with our resources in order to measure the time consumed in planning and following up treatment already decided. One series of interviews had to be discontinued, and a questionnaire yielded answers which could not be used, mainly because of our own difficulties in explaining our terms of reference to the doctors and nurses. Many of those questioned thought that 'planning and follow-up of treatment measures already decided upon' meant something quite different from what we intended. Some kind of measurement on the basis of observations is probably required in order to obtain reliable measurements.

The doctors and nurses clearly agree that planning and follow-up of treatment already decided are tasks which primarily consume the nurse's time. On the other hand, there is some disagreement in the opinions of nurses and doctors as to the extent of responsibility for planning and follow-up activities (see Fig. 7.8).

254

All the in-patient units at the hospital are manned in much the same way, regardless of the demands on the charge nurse with respect to functions such as patient planning. The allocation of ward secretaries and clerks has not been adapted to the demands which patient planning places on the staff. Table 7.10 shows that this condition can be regarded as inadequate for the demands of the situation; it reveals that when some charge nurses were asked to evaluate their needs for secretarial help (not the help they had when the question was asked), there is a very close relation between their answers and the results obtained earlier regarding the departments' degree of autonomy (see Table 5.20).

TABLE 7.10

Evaluations by a group of charge nurses as to their needs for secretarial help

Coefficient of dependency [10]	None	< Part-time	Part-time	> Part-time
0-0.24	3			
0.25-0.49	3	6		
0.50-0.74			3	
0.75-1.00				3

Our study of the hospital's hierarchy posed even more complicated problems of measurement, and we have refrained from doing anything more than a limited study of one clinical department.[11] Our expectation that roles would not be formally described was not met at all. There were job instructions for all the employees in a clinical department except the doctors, and the formal organisation structure was completely clear to almost all interviewees. However, a more detailed study of the real authority structure revealed large deviations from the formal plan and showed all the complexity and adaptability we had expected. When care of the acutely ill necessitates, almost anyone can ask anyone else for help, and the hierarchy for giving orders is nearly the opposite of the formal structure. The nursing auxiliary can 'give orders' to the nurse who 'gives orders' to the junior doctor who 'gives orders' to the department chief to act. This authority structure seems to be based on knowledge of the patient's needs. Another authority structure is based on medical competence (see Fig. 7.9). One exception is the on-call structure which supersedes the

255

normal structure. In other words, this structure is not the same during the day as at night.

We had many opportunities to make informal observations of how well the complicated authority structure functions at the hospital. The doctor often accepts a nurse's advice, and may even ask: 'What do you think we should do?' A moment later—in another matter—the authority structure changes completely, and the doctor gives the nurse distinct orders.

Consultations among doctors function well. On the basis of these observations, we shall formulate the hypothesis that formal and real conflicts are less common in a hospital than in industrial firms of the same size which are organised on the line-staff principle. We think that the most important reason why this highly complex authority structure functions well, and without conflicts, is that the hospital's employees have congruent goals. Of course, this hypothesis could not be measured in more than a few instances. But these cases were chosen with regard to the possibilities of finding incongruencies. Thus, for example, we tried to assess the staff's reactions to working methods and objectives in the long-term care department. This clinical department has recently been reorganised and has been assigned what are, in many respects, new goals. However, the scheme of methods and objectives which we constructed (Fig. 7.10) does not reveal any incongruencies.[12]

Areas of authority are classified fairly simply. These classifications govern relations within the clinical departments and between the departments and the service units. Thus, there are medical matters and medical service, for which orders can, in principle, be given only by doctors. This refers, for instance, to consultation with another doctor, eye and X-ray examinations, occupational therapy, or physiotherapy. The charge nurse can order routine tests, cleaning, supplies from the store-room, help from the maintenance unit, and similar matters.

Control within the hospital

Expectations

As described in chapter 4, there is no competitive market situation governing the relations between the hospital, the county authorities, and the patients. In addition, the county authorities and the patients are participants who are in a very weak position with respect to the hospital. In chapter 3 we described the hospital's continuing expansion, along with steadily increasing resources, during the last few decades. This implies that

256

rationalisation campaigns cannot be expected to be instituted by competition or crises and that the demand for efficiency is, thus, by no means one of the most important demands on the management or the employees at the hospital. Therefore, we expected both constant control of efficiency and, particularly, the organisational measures aimed at rationalisation to be deemed less urgent at the hospital than in an industrial firm.

In chapter 4 we said that the county authorities' most important demands on the hospital management involved acquiring personnel, keeping the hospital running and making effective use of the resources allocated to the hospital. Thus, we expected the management to use various means in an attempt to control factors such as absenteeism, staff turnover and the number of staff vacancies, as well as other factors which could be regarded as general measures of the hospital's ability to satisfy the county authorities' demands.

The absence of the market incentive makes it difficult to measure effectively results and efficiency within the hospital. Efficiency cannot be controlled on the basis of simple statistics. Instead, this has to be based on the care and attention exercised by supervisors in making decisions and on their professional values. This kind of decentralised control is also convenient since the hospital relies to such a large extent on relatively independent groups for carrying out its work (i.e. clinical departments). The great importance of medical decision-making (i.e. decisions on a particular course or method of treatment with respect to efficiency) also implies that department chiefs, who unquestionably have the greatest medical knowledge in the hospital, are alone in relation to their superiors, as well as their subordinates when it comes to evaluating and supervising efficiency. Therefore, we expected that, to the extent that employees at the hospital actually paid attention to the supervision and control of efficiency, they would systematically use the department chiefs for this task. We thought that this would take place through systematic attempts to influence the department chiefs' professional norms in order to make them more aware of their responsibility regarding the control of efficiency. We thus expected that there would be conscious efforts to preserve the autonomy of the departments, that the departments' chiefs would receive reports containing information about costs, volume of production and use of resources and that they would be given access to resources for studies and rationalisation.

The hospital is almost completely without economic reserves. If the annual budget is exceeded, an acute liquidity crisis occurs unless the county authorities intervene. Thus, we expected a great deal of attention to be devoted to the use of economic resources, for example, through

257

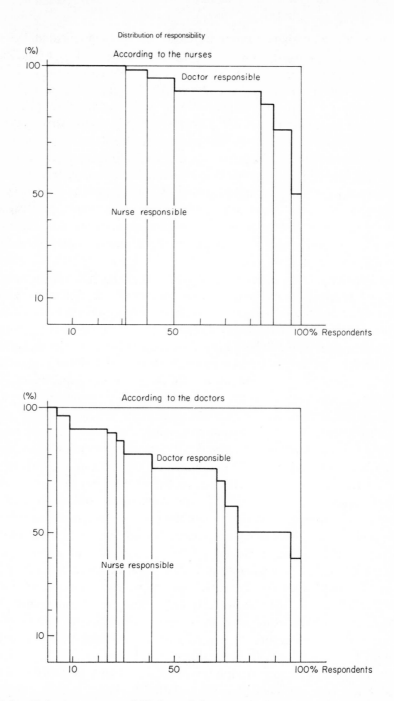

Distribution of responsibility

According to the nurses

Doctor responsible

Nurse responsible

According to the doctors

Doctor responsible

Nurse responsible

Fig. 7.8 Relative responsibilities of doctors and nurses for planning and follow-up clinical treatment measures already decided.

258

continual control of appropriations, which would be carried out with particular care towards the end of the budget year.

Measurements

Our expectation that little significance would be attached to the control of efficiency within the hospital was wholly realised. Owing to the importance of, and difficulty in evaluating the extent and weight of controls on efficiency, we used four complementary methods which all produced the same results.

First, we gathered information about the system of written reports within the hospital (Fig. 7.11). It turned out to be very difficult to obtain an overall picture of this system; there was no one at the hospital who had a comprehensive view of it. This means that the reporting system as a whole had never been reviewed. Many reports are late, and difficult to interpret—partly because there are no comparative figures. The situation with respect to the hospital's so-called operating accounts is particularly interesting. These accounts consist of an analysis of the hospital's operating costs classified according to origin and type. Cost-allocation account-

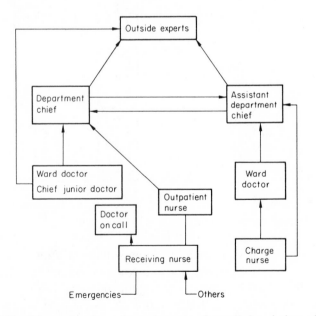

Fig. 7.9 The hierarchy in a department of medicine is based on medical competence.

259

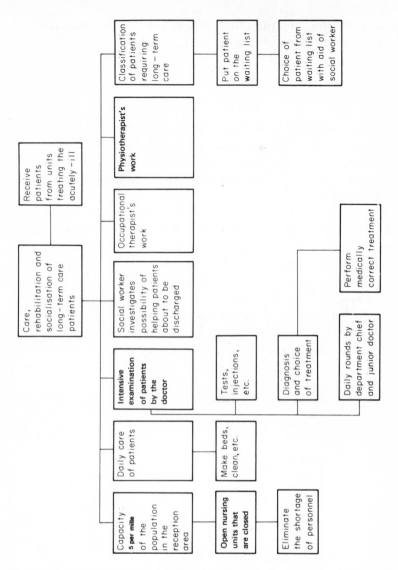

Fig. 7.10 Scheme of methods and objectives in the treatment of patients requiring long-term care.

ing presupposes extensive internal charges which, in some cases, are made on the basis of real measurements (e.g. of the extent to which various service units are utilised), and in others, on the basis of quotas. Operating accounts were introduced in 1963. The first cost report was presented in August 1964. The report for 1965 was presented in May 1966. In other words—these reports are not produced on time. The department chiefs

260

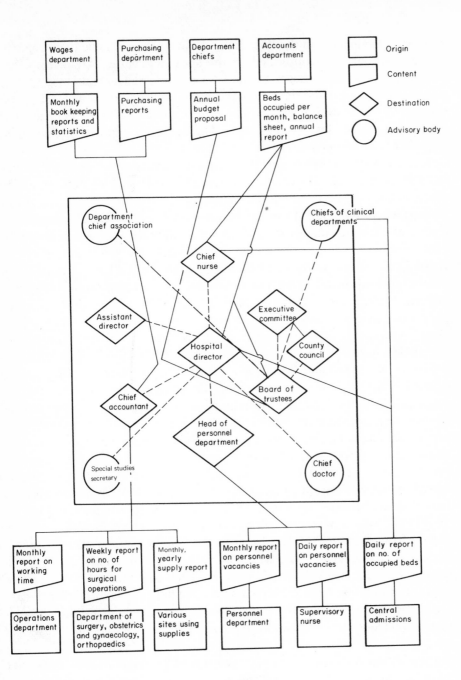

Fig. 7.11 System of reports at General Hospital.

261

and other top people in the hospital's administration receive these reports, and extracts are also published in the staff newspaper. Aside from this, however, no revisions seem to have been made at General Hospital (see below the accountants' statement about the auditing of the report). These reports have not even been discussed by the board of trustees. A critical member of the county council said, 'The operating report is a document intended for filing in a drawer'.

Second, a dozen persons in the hospital's management and the county council were asked: 'Do you have access to statistics which you can use to evaluate the performance and efficiency of the hospital as a whole, or of its various units?' Half those questioned said 'No' without reservation. Two said that they receive statistics on, for example, the average length of stay, number of admissions and surgical operations, but maintained that these figures are misleading and cannot be used for this kind of evaluation. Two others admitted to having received some reports, though they had not yet 'delved into the jungle of figures'. Yet two others had access to statistics, but when they gave examples of what they meant, they talked about completely irrelevant data (such as 'the age distribution of the population in the county').

Third, we investigated special actions taken at General Hospital to control efficiency. We took note of the amount of resources used for rationalisation, cuts in appropriations, and accounting. The resources allotted to rationalisation are limited, though much greater than they were a few years ago. The chief nurse and supervisory nurses thought that they could reserve about a third of their time for studying matters related to rationalisation. The operations and personnel departments were also involved in rationalisation projects to some extent. Moreover, the hospital has a special studies secretary. A general appropriation amounting to 30,000 cr., which was granted by the county council in 1965, was removed from the 1966 budget because the county council claimed that it wanted to concentrate resources for rationalisation in its own central organisation department. The budget for 1967 again includes this kind of appropriation. The total resources which the hospital devotes to rationalisation (including service from the county council's organisation department) thus amount to somewhere between three and four man years per year.

Rationalisation projects carried out, or in progress, during 1965 and 1966 are listed in Table 7.11. The main emphasis is on improved office routines and reduction of personnel in service functions and, to some extent, in nursing care. The largest projects involved shifting the storeroom accounting system to automatic data processing, and the introduc-

262

tion of preventive maintenance of machines. The latter was interrupted, however, because of the failure to gain support from a central committee. A study of the organisation of personnel services, carried out by a consultant, was very beneficial to the hospital. The consequences of this study were described in chapter 6.

The introduction of new routines for registering patients was a relatively minor project which nonetheless had large repercussions in the sense that two committees were formed to revise forms and routines for making appointments, the filing system for medical records, reception of patients, etc. A doctor also served on each of these committees. But these projects are not likely to be completed in the forseeable future unless more resources are allotted to them.

None of the people we interviewed could think of any instances in which requests for appropriations, or the personnel budget, were deliberately cut in order to enforce rationalisation. The way in which budget proposals are scrutinised was described earlier.

The hospital does not have its own internal auditing. On the other hand, the county council's accountants subject the hospital to fairly extensive auditing, primarily, examination of the accounts, with many spot checks on salary and other payments. The minutes of the meetings of the board of trustees are also examined. The accountants are probably the only people who have thus far tried to use the so-called operating accounts (cost statistics). The extent and content of the auditing at General Hospital is described in more detail in Table 7.12, which constitutes a survey of the items dealt with in the accountants' reports during a two-year period. Moreover, the table indicates that even the accountants found it difficult to come to any conclusions on the basis of operating accounts.

Fourth, we studied various opinions as to who was responsible for controlling efficiency. This phase was based on the assumption that a minimum prerequisite for controlling efficiency would consist of fairly common opinions of who was responsible. These common opinions were lacking at General Hospital to a large extent. The chief physician thought that it was the job of the hospital director. The hospital director thought that the chief nurse and supervisory nurses should control efficiency. The county council said that it was the board of trustees' responsibility, and a few members of the board felt that department chiefs were primarily responsible. The department chiefs, in turn, pointed their fingers at either the county authorities, the hospital director, or the chief nurse.

Our survey of the hospital's reporting system indicated that our expectations were at least partly realised in respect to the control exerted by

TABLE 7.11

Rationalisation projects carried out during 1965 and 1966

Area studied	Aim	Results	Analyst, and amount of time spent in the hospital
General organisational matters			
Organisation of personnel service	To survey personnel problems, their causes and propose action	Personnel department and programme for its activities established in 1966	Management consultant: approx. 5 man months; two work groups headed by department chiefs
Forms and routines for registering patients, making appointments, filing, reception, etc.	Uniform and rational routines	New routine for registering patients; the rest is still being worked on	Two committees consisting of the chief accountant, two department chiefs, the county council organisation assistant and a management consultant (begun in 1965)
Nursing care			
Methods and work schedule in the nursing units	More even work rhythm and simplification of nursing tasks	Some changes in the work schedule have been made, giving more convenient working hours	Chief nurse, supervisory nurses, and special studies secretary: approx. 1 man month
'Material studies'	Reduction in the no. of personnel and of costs through better equipment and use of disposable items	Recommendations for use of some disposable items carried out	Chief nurse and supervisory nurses: approx. 1/2 day/each week (in progress)
Medicines	Reduce costs	Work in progress	Pharmacy committee with a pharmacist as chairman: 3 meetings since April 1966

264

Office routines

Filing and secretaries in the X-ray department	Avoid increases in the need for personnel and appropriations	Aim achieved	Special studies secretary in cooperation with the county council organisation secretary: 2 man months
Medical secretaries in the department of surgery	Less overtime, with improved service to patients	Aim achieved	Special studies secretary: 1 man month
Store-room	Reduce no. of personnel and economise more in the store-room	Shift to ADP accomplished	Chief accountant and his assistants: approx. 1 man year
Medical statistics (diagnoses and surgical operations)	Reduce no. of personnel	Shift to ADP prepared	Chief accountant: 1 man month
Medical secretaries' pool	Determine the no. of personnel required	Work begun	County council organisation assistant in cooperation with special studies secretary

Service functions

Central baths	More even workload	Different departments use of bath facilities scheduled	Chief nurse and supervisory nurses. More extensive survey being prepared by county council organisation assistant: 2 man months
Internal transport	Simplification of methods; save work	Some recommendations made to the department of medicine	
Cleaning	Reduce no. of personnel and costs	Centralised cleaning introduced but expected reduction in personnel not yet achieved	Special studies secretary in cooperation with county council organisation assistant: 4 man months
Distribution of food	Reduce no. of personnel and costs	Experiments in central preparation of trays	Special studies secretary and consultant: approx. 2 man months

265

Table 7.11 (continued)

Area studied	Aim	Results	Analyst, and amount of time spent in the hospital
Preventive maintenance of machines	Reduce no. of personnel and costs	Study begun but shelved for the time being	1 man year
Other			
Building inspection	Reduce maintenance costs	Work in progress	Special studies secretary: 3 man months
Personnel directory	Simplify work in the personnel department	Directory compiled	Special studies secretary and personnel department: 3 man months
Bulletin boards	Better internal information	Uniform system being introduced	Chief nurse

266

the hospital management. The hospital director and the board of trustees receive reports from the chief nurse, the chief accountant, and the personnel department about the number of beds occupied in the nursing units and about personnel vacancies. A great deal of importance is attached to these reports and they often result in actions being taken. On the other hand, our expectation that statistics on staff turnover would also be reported was not met. This is probably due to the shortage of resources for compiling these statistics in the personnel department.

The expectation that the department chiefs would be influential in controlling efficiency was only partly realised. Of course, department heads check their nursing units daily when they make their rounds. These rounds take place regularly but do not last long. In addition, the department chiefs and their staff do not agree in some respects as to what should be included in this kind of supervision. There is no doubt that controls are aimed at supervising the application of professional norms, i.e. those covering hygiene, orderliness, and nursing methods but not waiting time, staff turnover, or use of resources. As far as we could tell, the hospital does not exert an active influence on these professional norms. Nor do department chiefs or other supervisors receive statistical reports which could be used as a basis for supervising production activities.

However, what surprised us most of all was that—contrary to our expectations—efforts were being made within the hospital to reduce the department chiefs' independence and responsibility. One important measure in this context was the reorganisation of the nursing staff, which then came under the authority of the chief nurse. This meant that the nursing units, and particularly, controls on efficiency in these units, became the responsibility of the supervisory nurses whose immediate superior is the chief nurse, who, in turn, does not come under the authority of the department chief. The establishment of central cleaning and central preparation of trays also helped to erode the independence of clinical departments. These actions are motivated primarily by the fact that they result in rationalisation made possible by coordination and use of common routines throughout the hospital.

During the course of our interviews, however, we often came across expressions of distrust as to the department chiefs' interest—and ability to interest themselves—in efficiency and rationalisation. Some interviewees implied that improvements could only be accomplished by relieving department chiefs of responsibility for them. Another aspect is that the department chiefs do not have resources available in their departments for rationalisation and development work. This line of reasoning is quite different from that usually advocated in industrial firms where product

267

TABLE 7.12
Auditing at General Hospital

Item	Accountant's action	Report or excerpts from minutes sent to the county health and medical services board	Actions resulted in (according to the accountant)
Collection of payments for patients' telephone bills		Uniform practice and simplified collection	+
Waiting time for admission		1. Actions to relieve General Hospital,	0
		2. Waiting lists should be taken into account when allocating resources,	0
		3. Reasons for waiting lists should be analysed,	0
		4. Patient should receive longer notice of admission	0
Inventory lists		Inventory lists should be kept	(+)
Collection of fees in X-ray department		Accounts should be rendered more rapidly and on a special form. Annual statements should be made.	+
Medical secretaries		Not advisable for doctor to pay extra salary to the secretaries on account of collection of patient's fees. County council should provide office staff to do this.	0

Insurance	After private contact with the hospital director, insurance against water damage was recommended.	
	Survey of the various kinds of insurance.	(+)
Accounting procedures	Memorandum presented to the hospital director and agreement reached that:	
	1. Bills amounting to less than 1 cr. will not be made out,	+
	2. Pay telephones will be installed in personnel residences,	0
	3. Petty-cash drawer possibly to be introduced,	(+)
	4. Purchase of fish to be watched carefully.	+
Personnel planning for long-term care	Expansion plans should be adapted to available personnel	0
Purchase of works of art for the long-term care department	Previous appropriations not used	0
Operating budget 1963	1. Uniform rules	+
Operating budget 1964 (lack of uniformity in accounting principles made comparisons and interpretation impossible)	2. Continual 'controls on effectiveness' through reports on the length of waiting lists	0
	3. A coordinating committee should be appointed.	+

+ Proposal carried out
(+) Proposal being studied
0 No action taken

269

organisation, divisionalisation, and similar actions are aimed at creating units which are as independent as possible, enabling each manager to become fully responsible for the efficiency and results of his unit.

We tried to find out about controls on appropriations by interviewing those at the hospital responsible for auditing, and influential persons within the hospital and county council. The normal accounting which is done at the hospital is aimed at ensuring that the hospital's budget is not exceeded; this auditing is very simple and always up to date. The hospital's budget covers about ninety items, and the accounting involves classification of costs according to these ninety accounts. Around the tenth of each month the hospital director receives a report on the status of appropriations on the last day of the preceding month. Capital accounts are checked in terms of the book value of expenditures, as well as advance orders. This is because a long time often elapses between a binding decision to incur an expense, and the actual date of payment. Another reason is that past (unfortunate) experience has shown that construction costs rise, and turn out to be higher than anticipated. Costs are also affected to a large extent because repairs and maintenance are often postponed.

In addition, the county council keeps a close watch on General Hospital's costs as the end of the year approaches. The county council expects a forecast before 1 November as to whether the budget may be exceeded. If it looks as if it may, additional appropriations are requested; this might occur at any time of the year. However, most requests for additional funds are made towards the end of the budget year, especially in November and December. If other accounts are expected to yield a budget surplus, then a redistribution is made. Otherwise, additional appropriations are granted. Neither the board of trustees, the health and medical services board, nor the executive committee attach much importance to—or even discuss—the fact that the budget is exceeded. In 1965, General Hospital made six requests—one of them large—for additional funds amounting to 3 per cent of the total operating budget. The corresponding figures in 1964 were four requests and 1 per cent of the operating budget. All requests were granted.

The main reason why our expectations about controls on appropriations were not met is that we completely misjudged the hospital's economic situation. General Hospital has no financial reserves to fall back on. This means that the county authorities need greater reserves than might otherwise be expected. At the end of 1965, the county council had 20.8 million cr. in various contingency and surplus funds, corresponding to 11.3 per cent of the county's operating and capital budget for 1966.

270

Notes

[1] Source: G. Biörck, 'Journalens uppgifter och utformning' (Purposes and Content of Medical Records), *Svenska Läkartidningen 61:16*, 1964, p. 1309.

[2] An experienced doctor, however, made the following comment in an earlier version of the report. 'This is typical nurses' nonsense. These are things every doctor knows, even if the nurse imagines that she can tell the doctor a thing or two. Things like this don't belong in this book.'

[3] Previous salary systems for doctors influenced the allocation of resources between in-patient and outpatient care in ways that are no longer applicable since the introduction of the new fee system (see chapter 4).

[4] See note 3.

[5] The hospital pharmacist automatically selects the cheapest drug if there are 'synonyms'.

[6] By mistake, this question was put to department chiefs only.

[7] See note 3 above.

[8] In checking our manuscript, a department chief objected to this expression of the county council's view of education. But it is probably correct that doctors often find it difficult to get away from their daily obligations.

[9] When we discussed this matter with doctors and nurses at the hospital, they maintained that knowledge obsolescence is a more serious problem for nurses than doctors. This may be true, but 82 per cent of the nurses did not respond to this question, so it is impossible to interpret the results.

[10] This is the coefficient of dependency for in-patient and outpatient care (the quotient of the cost of external services and internal wages; see chapter 5).

[11] We discovered an important inadequacy in organisation theory when we tried to measure the authority structure. Measurements of this kind have only been carried out in a few cases and the methods used are described very sketchily.

[12] These methods of measurement and investigation are based on theories described in more detail in C. Wallroth, 'An Analysis of Means-end Structures', *Acta Sociologica* 11, 1968, pp. 110f. (SIAR-24).

271

8 A Contribution to the Debate

We began this study of a medium-sized Swedish hospital by describing the conditions under which the hospital management works. These conditions were summarised under two headings: 'the hospital's participant relations' and 'the hospital's production system'. An analysis of the hospital's administration appeared in chapter 7.

Our original intention was to let the reader draw his own conclusions after we had described these conditions. Our primary aim was to assess the possibilities of making a systematic analysis of the hospital's administration on the basis of propositions derived from different parts of organisation theory, and some general standardised concepts. But as our work progressed, the idea of extending our study emerged. The answers we obtained from the question 'Is the hospital's administration adapted to the demands of the situation?' should possibly be formulated as direct hypotheses about the relation between suggested administrative and organisational changes and the hospital's effectiveness. These statements would apply primarily to General Hospital in Industry Town, and to the extent that conditions there are representative of Swedish hospitals in general, the propositions could also refer to the group as a whole. From this point of view, our study could be regarded as an exploration culminating in a number of hypotheses.

When the decision to formulate these hypotheses was made, the question immediately arose as to how they could be tested. Could we convince the county council in question to implement changes in order to assess the validity of the hypotheses? Perhaps this was not completely impossible, but a single experiment involving so many simultaneous changes would cause enormous methodological problems, especially in interpreting the effects. Thus, we decided to carry out more unconventional and less expensive tests of our hypotheses by having employees of General Hospital and the county council, as well as hospital experts in central agencies and in the rest of the county, scrutinise our proposals.

These proposals are generally derived from the debate on hospital administration. Certain details of some of our suggestions may be original. However, our primary aim was not to make original proposals but to summarise the most important changes which—if carried out simultaneously—could be expected to increase effectiveness at General Hospital.

273

Thus, the most important aspect of this process is the *choice* of proposals or hypotheses. This implies that it is just as important to observe which proposals are included, as it is to discern which have been omitted. It should also be noted that expectations as to increased effectiveness refer to the simultaneous execution of all proposals. If only isolated proposals are implemented, the results, in most instances, will be limited improvements in effectiveness, or perhaps even impairment.

Execution of this phase of our study

A draft of our report served as a basis for discussions of these hypotheses. Five seminars were held for this purpose, and employees of General Hospital and the county council participated in two. Experts in hospital administration employed in central agencies and other county councils participated in the other three. The way in which these seminars were conducted varied a great deal—which meant that it turned out to be meaningless to analyse the answers statistically. Those who took part in the seminars were given a copy of the report in advance. The author acted as chairman, and the report was discussed and explained. A list of the hypotheses presented below was also distributed to the seminar participants for discussion in smaller groups. Minutes were made of most of the discussions.

The participants in some of the seminars were asked to evaluate the proposals according to a five-point scale. Before evaluating the hypotheses, they were given the following written instructions, which were also explained orally by the author:

On the basis of your own experience, evaluate the measures proposed in the list of hypotheses, using the following scale:

I think that the measures proposed would contribute to
5 = increasing the hospital's effectiveness significantly
4 = increasing the hospital's effectiveness to some extent
3 = neither increasing nor decreasing the hospital's effectiveness
2 = decreasing the hospital's effectiveness to some extent
1 = decreasing the hospital's effectiveness significantly

Please observe that:

$$\text{Effectiveness} = \frac{\text{Sum total of needs satisfied through the hospital's activities}}{\text{Sum total of economic and personnel contributions made in the hospital}}$$

274

Each proposal should be evaluated in its entirety.

Please write down personal comments, for instance, by mentioning the most important advantages and disadvantages related to various subproposals. When evaluating each proposal, it should be assumed that all other proposals would be implemented simultaneously. Evaluate *all the proposals*, including those whose effects you find difficult to predict.

The participants were not chosen at random from a large population but were selected systematically with respect to their interest in hospital administration. (This is another reason why statistical analysis of the answers was impossible.) Thus, the following discussion of our hypotheses contains only qualitative interpretations of the experts' evaluations. Important comments are also cited.

There are reservations in interpreting the results. Although the participants in the seminars were not selected with regard to any special expectations about their attitudes, I had considerable influence on the choice of participants in two of the seminars. Thus, it is not unlikely that I, and my advisers, classified as experts persons with experience and values similar to ours. However, an even more important factor is that I began all seminars by presenting a resumé of the report. Then I presented the proposals and, at least briefly, gave reasons for them. This implies, of course, that I consciously tried to influence the participants.

Most of the discussions were held in small groups of three to seven persons. In other words, the opinions described below are common to these groups as a whole. However, the participants' written comments were handed to me individually. If these reservations are kept in mind, it should be possible to regard the following account as a contribution to the debate.

Preliminary list of hypotheses

1. Measures which alter relations with county authorities or the main organisation of the hospital

(a) Either or both of the following two measures should be taken: Either the county council should be given much greater resources for research, including medical expertise, or the hospital management (board of trustees, chief of medical staff, and hospital director) should be given significantly greater responsibility and freedom of

275

action. (In the propositions below, it is assumed that the latter alternative is chosen.)

The experts subscribed wholeheartedly to this hypothesis. A common reaction was that they wanted to implement these measures. The following was proposed in various ways:

The goals of different medical units should be formulated on a central level and on the county council level, which requires some reconstruction. Other decisions should in principle be decentralised as far down as possible, i.e. on the hospital level.

In all the groups in which this proposal was discussed, the participants thought that the budget should be used as an instrument to achieve the amount of central planning and local independence desired.

I think that the hospital's management should have more freedom of action, but this cannot be attained unless another budget system is introduced.

We shall return to this problem later.

(b) The executive subcommittee of the board of trustees should receive more resources, primarily in the form of an increase in salary and freedom from other duties for the chief physician and chairman of the board.

In general, the experts were in favour of this proposal, though a large group was indifferent and thought that it would not lead to either improvement or impairment of conditions. This was also reflected in some of the comments.

The chief of the medical staff should retain his medical activity. Do we really need a board of trustees?
One prerequisite is that doctors receive special education and training in hospital administration both during and after medical school.

In addition, the experts repeatedly pointed out that an increase in resources is not the same as greater economic compensation. Nor is it cer-

276

tain that increased economic compensation has anything to do with the contributions of the chairman and the chief of medical staff.

(c) The department chiefs' association at General Hospital should be authorised as an agent for consultation and information exchange between hospital management and department chiefs.

All the participants agreed with his proposal, though some of them said that such authorisation could limit opportunities for informal deliberations and lead to 'more red tape'. Others wanted to discuss the composition of the department chiefs' association. Two experts thought that junior doctors should also be represented. One said:

If departmental blocs are created, the association should consist of the hospital director and the bloc chiefs—although one person would be appointed to head the association.

But another said:

The way things are now the answer to this question is yes, but it becomes more doubtful if the bloc system were introduced.

(d) The seventeen clinical departments in the hospital should be combined into approximately four clinical blocs headed by a department chief (to whom the other department chiefs in the bloc would be subordinate). The bloc chiefs would be appointed for a limited time, have greater administrative powers, and fewer medical duties. The salary for this job would clearly indicate status superior to that of the clinical department chiefs. The division into clinical blocs could be adapted to the experience and interests of the chiefs.

Most of the participants were in favour of this hypothesis, though quite a few objected. There were many comments, which can be roughly classified as follows:

Views on the bloc chief's authority
Views on the bloc chief's duties
Necessary prerequisites for the reform

Most of those who were dubious about this proposal said they had misgivings about the bloc chief's authority. The following comments illustrate this point.

The bloc chief's authority:

A specialist will not accept a bloc chief whose speciality is different. This will only lead to dissension.

I don't believe in lesser status for the bloc chief as compared with a department chief. Teaching hospitals might be an exception.

It's doubtful whether the bloc chief would have the authority intended. The duties of the chief of the medical staff should be increased instead, to achieve the degree of coordination required.

I don't think this kind of an arrangement would meet difficulties. He could be a junior doctor, of course, and then some difficulties could present themselves in cooperation with more highly educated colleagues.

If a doctor is to retain his status, he has to have complete professional knowledge and still be able to fulfil his medical duties, e.g. perform an ear operation. A technical administrator doesn't have to be capable of turning a screw when he becomes boss.

The bloc chief's duties (the following statements reflect the degree of confusion about these):

It's unreasonable to suggest that another colleague should become acquainted with four different specialties.

The bloc chief's duties are obscure.

Would the beds be at this bloc chief's disposal?

The bloc chief would be some kind of a secretary or errand boy for the department chief.

Prerequisites for the reform—education:

The experts did not think that the reform could be accomplished without some special education for the doctors. And they were doubtful as to whether this could be obtained.

Then the doctors would have to study administration and managerial economics.

The principle is excellent. The problem is that there is no suitable education at the present time.

278

This is a purely theoretical idea which could not be achieved given the way in which medical care is organised in Sweden today.

The possibility of producing this kind of administrative physician is too far-fetched.

(e) The bloc chief should be given large freedom of action, such as in choosing between employing new personnel or in buying outside services. (See also 2a)

Half the participants approved, and half disapproved of this hypothesis. One group came to the conclusion that this proposal was a necessary consequence of the preceding one. Another thought that there had to be some restrictions. The physicians (including several department chiefs at General Hospital) thought that the department chief should not be by-passed in such an important matter. One expert in hospital administration did not think that the proposal was suitable given the present personnel situation, since the blocs would compete for scarce resources.

(f) The complexity of the cooperation between different individuals and units should not be eliminated even if it means double authority. On the other hand, everyone should be aware of who is boss for whom, and of the significance of the position of chief, especially in terms of responsibility for employee appraisal and personnel welfare.

In general, this proposal was approved, though a large group thought that these measures would not mean much. This was primarily because the suggestion did not involve changes in present conditions. A mixed group from General Hospital came to the conclusion that, even though they were in favour of the proposal, the distribution of roles and responsibility had to be made very clear.

(g) Patients who put pressure on bottlenecks at General Hospital (such as the department chiefs) and who do not require General Hospital's resources should be transferred to other medical institutions. The most important example is that only referral patients should be treated in most departments.

This proposal was strongly approved of—almost without exception. However, it was pointed out that there would be considerable practical difficulties in carrying it out in view of present conditions.

The gist of the matter is to create these 'other medical institutions'; group practices are not democratic; long-term care has only recently been given priority for expansion.

Another group pointed out that this proposal could possibly be put into effect in the county where General Hospital is located. But this cannot be done everywhere. 'Rural areas present considerable problems.' Two department chiefs were opposed to the proposal on the grounds that 'the patient-screening function was not taken into account. This had to be the responsibility of the department chiefs.'

(h)   An admissions unit for emergencies should possibly be set up in every clinical bloc which would be designed to allow for a 50 per cent capacity reserve. The admissions unit would serve as a buffer between the fluctuating patient flow and the nursing units.

This proposal also met approval, though practical difficulties were pointed out. Some experts felt that the proposal could not be achieved in all instances, e.g. for all maternity cases, premature babies, etc. There would also have to be a separate admissions unit for infectious diseases.
   Others wanted to extend this hypothesis even further and thought that a single admissions department for the whole hospital would be the most suitable. This would facilitate cooperation between the clinical blocs. One expert added:

The admissions unit should be given this overcapacity at the same time that pressure is exerted on the way patients are treated in the clinical departments. Otherwise the interim unit will become rapidly filled and this implies inconsistent and poor treatment.

(i)   A transitional nursing unit with considerable overcapacity under normal conditions should be established and function as a buffer between the hospital and other institutions.

The experts' opinions on this proposal are very similar to their attitudes towards the preceding hypothesis. They approve of the proposal but point

280

out the difficulties involved in carrying it out. One group summarised their point of view by saying 'The idea is right, but it's impossible today.' Attitudes towards carrying out this proposal are reflected in the following statements.

The rehabilitation department should be expanded and become a transition department for helping patients readjust to their jobs and life outside the hospital. One of the county council's most important tasks is planning for the expansion of long-term care.

We used to have post-hospital care and we miss it a great deal now.

As things are now, this kind of transition department could easily become a purely custodial unit.

Unfortunately, however, the overcapacity would be utilised fully so that problems would merely be transferred from one clinical department to another. Compare this to the present dilemma in long-term care.

It's worth a try. This would probably depend on the way nursing units are set up in the future, that is if specialties are done away with and patients are classified according to difficult, easy, or day care.

The idea seems good in principle. But where will the boundaries lie? Who will be medically responsible for the patients who are moved out? Patients in transitional unit would run the risk of getting stuck there. In addition, it's unpleasant to have to move patients often.

(j) A reserve of mobile personnel including doctors, nurses and other nursing personnel, who are more qualified and paid higher salaries than average, would be recruited and placed at the disposal of the hospital management to be assigned to departments or units when acute personnel shortage arise. Departments which make use of this reserve would be charged a price significantly higher than the normal cost of personnel.

Most of the experts were also in favour of this hypothesis. One group felt that it would be advantageous to district physicians, and others who might be in need of comprehensive practical experience, to become part of this mobile reserve. However, some experts were opposed to this hypothesis mainly because of the difficulties involved in finding sufficiently qualified doctors and nurses.

281

Versatile personnel such as this just don't exist. I can't picture doctors and nurses having this much flexibility.

These objections were also discussed by a mixed group of experts who concluded, 'Yes, give it a try.'

2. Measures aimed at influencing the goal perception or information system of members of the organisation

(a) The chief of a clinical bloc should have a flexible budget, i.e. a total appropriation which could be adjusted upwards or downwards depending on the amount and quality of care administered by his bloc. The chief would be free to use the total appropriation in any way he deems suitable. He would also be able to use some of the surplus for research or personnel benefits.

The experts were not unanimous in their opinions about this proposal, and their many comments varied a great deal. The group that seemed to have the best insight into the problem stated:

The decisive factor is the extent to which the quantity and quality of care can be measured. We feel it is imperative that an experiment in making these kinds of measurements be carried out as soon as possible.

Several objections reflect a lack of confidence in the way the bloc chief would use his new-found freedom:

All extra funds would go to research. The idea is correct, but there aren't very many people who could manage it.
There is a risk that certain departments would become scapegoats.

(b) The present 'piecework' salaries of doctors should be replaced by a system based on work and merit ratings.

The experts were not unanimous in their opinions about this proposal. However, 10 out of 13 department chiefs at General Hospital did approve it, and thought that it would result in an increase in effency. Two of the groups did not think that they were in a position to discuss the matter

282

because their members included representatives for employers and employees. In other words, they were afraid to make statements which could be used in future negotiations. The most important objection was that the proposed change in the salary system would result in decreased work efforts in outpatient care.

Yes, this proposal should be put into effect. The purpose, of course, is to limit outpatient care. But where should patients who need care go? Some kind of norms have to be established with respect to the physician's normal performance.

The way things are now, doctors should receive some kind of compensation to stimulate outpatient care.

The practical preconditions for executing this proposal will exist when all forms of outpatient care have been expanded in the future (perhaps in about twenty years!)

(c) The salary system for other personnel, which is based on 'salary levels' should be replaced by a more flexible system based on work and merit ratings.

Here, too, many of the experts did not think that they were in a position to evaluate the proposal.

This has to do with sensitive union matters. Personally, I think the wisest thing for me to do is supress my desires to participate in the debate, keep my mouth shut, and let others settle these matters.

The experts who did have something to say about this proposal were generally unfamiliar with salary matters.

(d) Measures should be taken to lessen status differentiation, though professional awareness should not be lessened, but augmented in the process. More education and examination of medical personnel, and opportunities for a career in the hospital (where the hospital would pay for further education) are examples of measures which could be taken.

None of those questioned opposed this proposal. However, some of the groups disposed of the matter quickly by concluding:

283

We think a lessening of status differentiation should be taken for granted.

One respondent wanted to point out that a decrease in status differentiation involved certain undesirable consequences:

Without status differentiation, one of the incentives for further education and choice of a demanding career would be eliminated. And don't forget that a chief's responsibility in critical situations requires absolute subordination.

(e) The hospital should actively utilise different professional organisations to create and influence professional norms and ideals. Leadership requirements should be included as important elements in the knowledge of 'a good nurse' or 'a good doctor'.

All respondents approved of this proposal. A small group did not think that conditions would be either improved or worsened by it. Some members of this group pointed out that it would be difficult to make changes in professional norms and ideals. They were also dubious as to the definition of the professional ideal contained in the proposal.

The proposal is good but it doesn't solve the problem and it's even more difficult to create a whole corps of 'saints'.
This is a good suggestion, but very difficult to put into effect nowadays. The organisation has only one interest: higher salaries.
It's obvious that someone can be a 'good doctor' or a 'good nurse' and still be a rather poor supervisor.

Two of the groups became very involved with this question and strongly emphasised the importance of the proposal. It was pointed out that many doctors and nurses do not adhere to professional norms and ideals.

(f) The quality of care in the departments should be measured regularly on the basis of statistics and the patients' attitudes. The latter type of subjective data should carry as much weight as statistics based on objective data on the results of treatment.

This was one of the proposals which was criticised the most. Of course, a

284

few experts were positive towards it, though just as many thought it would tend to make conditions worse. The idea objected to the most was that of using patients' attitudes to measure the quality of care in the departments. Some of the statements are summarised as follows:

Patients' subjective opinions do not mean that care was good or bad. Of course, if a hospital is going to be evaluated as if it were a hotel, then the patient's attitudes are more important. But how are you going to measure a patient's attitude? Isn't there a risk that patients will be wooed?

However, the most positive seminar group expressed itself carefully:

We're somewhat afraid of the phrase 'that subjective data should carry as much weight as objective data'. When data are obtained in this way, they have to be evaluated judiciously and taken for what they're worth.

(g) Cost reports which include the costs of internal services should be distributed on a monthly basis, and ten days after the end of the month at the latest, to all chiefs who are in a position to influence costs. These cost reports should be coordinated with statistics on 'production volume' and 'quality measurements'. Every chief should be instructed to discuss the cost reports with his subordinates.

The experts all agreed with the hypothesis that 'cost reporting and cost follow-ups are necessary for the other proposals to function'. But one group which discussed this matter very carefully had a more cautious view:

We're very sceptical towards the value of cost reports, especially with the way costs appear in the operating budget at present, with rather artificial allocations for indirect costs. It might be possible to make some kind of cost reports convincing in order to stimulate a certain amount of cost awareness. But we think it's very difficult as long as the reports are not combined—as it says here—with some measurement of, or statistics on, production and quality. In other words, the significance or value of cost reports would be increased many times over if they could be set in relation to results in some way. What we would like to see most is a higher degree of result and efficiency awareness rather than an increase in cost awareness.

285

(h) Written guidelines should be set up in each clinical department or bloc with respect to admissions criteria, methods of treatment, medical records, behaviour towards patients, and other matters which should be discussed in principle and where more experienced employees could guide the younger ones or where uniform behaviour would be required.

The evaluations of this proposal were interesting because most respondents were very positive and a minority was decidedly critical. The latter said:

It is dangerous to paralyse action because of rigid directives. Written guidelines are not suited to every department, personnel category, individual employee, etc.

One expert said he had thought about this question quite a lot and had discussed it with several others, including two professors of medicine. He stated:

There were many written instructions in one professor's department, whereas the other had more or less avoided them. I don't think the latter department is less effective than the former. It might be that some other form of indoctrination and control system has been established in the latter department, thus rendering written instructions superfluous. A set of the type of instructions you have in mind may be extremely valuable, but it can also become complicated very quickly. The main thing is that either the department chief himself, or one of his assistants, takes constant responsibility for this task.

A mixed group of experts said they agreed with the idea expressed in the hypothesis, but they suggested something quite different:

We'd like to emphasise that from many points of view it would be suitable for some higher authority to set up these guidelines—whether it be the National Board of Health and Welfare, the county council, the medical services board, or someone else. Their directives could guide the departments in their work. We do not think that the departments should be forced to adhere to guidelines; they should be able to retain a high degree of freedom. In any case, it would be appropriate to formulate these guidelines on a relatively high level.

286

3. Measures which create increased or improved resources for development

(a) The budget of each bloc should contain an additional margin for development and rationalisation. The chiefs of the clinical blocs should be free to determine the extent to which they make use of these resources. For example, they should be able to choose between employing their own experts, purchasing services from the chief nurse, or using consultants from outside the hospital. The chief of a clinical bloc should be held responsible for the extent to which he employs personnel.

In general, this proposal was approved, though there were a few objections. The main reason why this proposal led to several lively discussions is that a number of changes had already taken place in this area, e.g. the establishment of the chief nurse/supervisory nurse system and the expansion of rationalisation expertise under the jurisdiction of the county council. This proposal served as a catalyst for a number of views on existing conditions.

(b) The supervisory nurses should become subordinated to the chiefs of the clinical blocs. More resources should be allotted to the chief nurse, and she should become a central consulting authority in matters related to organisation and methods. Doctors should also be part of this consultant activity on a full- or part-time basis.

The experts were in favour of changes in the direction indicated by this hypothesis, though they suggested different variations. Four statements are worth quoting:

All this is highly uncertain with respect to the chief nurse. I'd rather see this institution disappear. It should be replaced by a physician responsible for rationalisation, or by a technician.

I think each bloc chief, or possibly each department chief, should have someone at his disposal who could achieve the necessary changes.

The charge nurse would have to be more specialised, be promoted, and more highly educated. I think that small clinical departments could consider letting charge nurses act in this capacity.

This is a dubious matter. In this case, the chief nurse should be

287

given the title of organisation assistant or head of the planning department. Therefore, the whole question seems unclear.

(c) Department chiefs, assistant department chiefs or junior physicians should be granted leave of absence when they are called on to participate in administrative or organisational research for the county council, the hospital management, or the chiefs of the clinical blocs. These research studies should be regarded as equivalent to medical work in terms of merits for salary determination and promotion.

This was one of the proposals which the experts approved of the most. However, it should be kept in mind that this opinion is somewhat biased because the doctors who participated in the discussions were highly medically and scientifically oriented. Two of the groups also pointed out that implementation of the proposal would 'run into great difficulties with respect to those who currently perform these studies'. Others maintained, however, that there is already a tendency in this direction.

4. Measures which lead to better planning

(a) Long-term plans, including plans for development and rationalisation, should be drawn up for each clinical bloc and for the hospital as a whole. The most important—and not the least controversial—projects should be given priority in these plans.

This proposal received the strongest support from the experts. No objections were made.

(b) Special measures should be taken for patient groups which require coordination between several departments. The chiefs of the clinical blocs should be responsible for carrying out these measures. Possible measures include conferences about patients or groups of patients, written guidelines for coordination between departments, or the appointment of special 'coordinating physicians' who could be responsible for coordinating follow-up visits and contacts with referring doctors.

There were mixed opinions about this proposal. The idea of a 'coordinating physician' seemed to cause the most doubt. On the other hand, most

288

of the experts approved of conferences about patients or groups of patients—and pointed out that this already takes place to some extent. One group thought that there was a connection between this hypothesis and the responsibility and right to admit patients to a clinical department. They had nothing against experimenting with a system whereby one doctor would act as chief, and another as coordinating physician. The latter would hold conferences, discussions, etc. to direct patients to the place where he thought they should be treated.

Another possible experiment would involve dispensing with the present system of department chiefs who have the right to admit patients, and instead, have a number of beds available to the organisation as a whole. The coordinating physician would then assign patients to a bed where a medical specialist would take charge of treatment.

(c) Charge nurses in units which are highly dependent on service units should be helped by a qualified assistant. This assistant's most important task would be to plan schedules and to follow up measures which are taken outside the department in accordance with the doctor's or nurse's instructions. The planning assistant should receive special education in how the hospital functions, as well as training in the various service units he or she will be working with.

In general, the experts agreed with this proposal. Some, however, were critical and felt that 'the nurse is the best person to be in charge of planning'.

5. *Measures which improve supervision or personnel conditions*

(a) One of the following two measures should be taken. Either the county council should hire a qualified personnel expert, or the personnel department at General Hospital should be made responsible for the hospital's relations with its staff. Important principles which should be included are: the salary system, division of work between different professional groups and more extensive recruitment of foreign manpower. Of course, the person made responsible for these matters should consult and cooperate with the central employer organisation (the Association of County Councils), the National Board of Health and Welfare, the labour market authorities, etc.

289

Most of the experts approved of this proposal and generally recommended the latter alternative which implied that the local personnel departments would gain more responsibility. However, objections were also raised, mainly of the type: 'What would happen if every small hospital began to do this kind of work?'

A group of experts with a great deal of knowledge about conditions also presented a detailed description of the reasons why they thought that personnel services should be centralised at the county council.

> Certain matters require common responsibility in the area as a whole. Examples are personnel forecasts, other measures aimed at promoting recruitment, and in general, expansion of the recruitment base. This also applies to general educational measures aimed at supplying the various personnel resources which might be needed. One example of this is the recruitment of foreign manpower. Therefore, we don't think each individual hospital should become involved in things like this. We believe this should be taken care of centrally, as it is now.

(b) The responsibility for personnel administrative measures aimed at guaranteeing a supply of staff should mainly be assumed by the chiefs of the clinical blocs. Those chiefs who so wish should be able to appoint a colleague as head of the unit's personnel. The central personnel service should coordinate activities, and give service when called on to help supply personnel.

Most of the experts, including department chiefs and others, were definitely critical of this proposal. They all gave the same reason for their criticism. They fear competition and a lack of coordination between the blocs. The following statement is typical:

> If the hospital is going to be organised according to blocs, then the chiefs of these blocs have the primary responsibility for rational management and administration of the personnel and material resources at the disposal of the bloc as a whole. This means that the chief has to be prepared to take the responsibility for many personnel administrative measures. But if this went so far that the chief could independently hire personnel and execute all the functions now carried out by the personnel department, then the hospital would end up with four separate personnel departments. A bloc which had control of personnel matters could even turn away

290

applicants because it didn't need them. On the other hand, we would like to point out other personnel administrative measures, particularly those related to personnel welfare. There are so many personnel administrative matters which are directly linked to specific organisational areas that certain kinds of hiring can never be concentrated in a personnel department as long as it remains outside the activity going on within the bloc.

(c) A five year plan for personnel supply should be made, and coordinated with the general plan for the hospital as a whole.

The experts all agreed with this proposal. But some maintained that personnel planning already takes place. This reflects the fact that they do not regard personnel planning as it is interpreted in modern business administration.[1]

(d) The hospital should not be expanded in the future unless the supply of personnel is assured and the hospital can retain a certain amount of freedom with regard to recruitment.

All the experts approved of this proposal, though they expressed a different opinion in some of their comments.

This proposal should be linked to the preceding one. It's one thing to make a personnel plan. You draw up an educational plan and it might even be in agreement with the general overall plan. But no one can claim that these measures ensure a supply of personnel. It's very popular nowadays to say that we should refrain from building hospitals because we won't get enough personnel anyway. But this is not a static situation—it's really a matter of how we've decided to act. For instance, if we have decided to build a new hospital or a new clinical department, we should also see to it that personnel are educated and recruited.

Expansion is often a prerequisite for obtaining personnel. If expansions are not carried out, then employees don't come. It might be possible to realise this proposal with new building methods and new types of medical units for all kinds of care.

291

(e)   The personnel department at General Hospital should be given more resources and the personnel manager should be more highly qualified.

To the extent that conditions at General Hospital were known in this matter, the experts agreed with this proposal. Otherwise, they said that it was difficult to have any opinion.

(f)   Through information to employees, consultation with the unions and education of supervisors, checks on slack (i.e. absence, promptness and breaks) should be legitimised as a management task.

The respondents (even those who were supervisors themselves!) unanimously approved this proposal. However, one group that carefully discussed this matter stated:

We fully agree that certain things must be done. The question is how. We have discussed whether this could be done as an experiment, but it seems rather strange in a hospital to say that now we're going to perform an experiment which means that 'employees should be on time, not take long breaks and do their work the way everyone has assumed that they or their chiefs do'.

(g)   A department chief or assistant department chief in each clinical bloc should be made responsible for planning further education (including that of doctors). Each employee should have a plan for his or her further education.

Most of the experts were enthusiastically in favour of this proposal. But some doubted whether a clinical chief or assistant department chief could assume this responsibility.

We think this seems like an enormous task. Of course, there have to be educational plans, but planning has to cover groups and not individuals on certain levels. We agree that the chief of a clinical bloc should be made responsible for this, and that he should be assisted in this task.

292

6. Measures which strengthen the patient's position

(a) A central agency for patient information and patient service should be established, possibly linked with the job of chief social worker, who could act as adviser to the hospital's management, departments, and chiefs of the clinical blocs. The responsibility for patient information and service should be decentralised.

There were mixed opinions about this proposal. The main objection involved the establishment of a central agency for patient information and service, but this may have been due to a misunderstanding. Objections centred on the fact that considerable competence would be required to handle the patients' medical problems. However, this was not what we intended by the proposal, and the small number of comments probably indicates that this matter was not considered especially important.

(b) Patients should be given more opportunity to make complaints above the level of the department chief. For example, a physician could be employed as patient ombudsman with the task of hearing complaints and reporting to the board of trustees. The patient ombudsman should not work in the hospital; instead he should work in outpatient care, in another county, etc.

Opinion for, and against, this proposal was about equally divided and was based on several kinds of arguments. Some of the experts pointed out that the county health officer already acts as a kind of patient ombudsman. Others felt that patients can complain to the National Board of Health and Welfare, the chairman of the board of trustees, or others in the county council. Still others said that even if there might be some advantages to this proposal: 'What doctor would want to act as patient ombudsman before his colleagues?'

Note

[1] See Cox, A., Margulies, A., and Söderlund, J., *Personalplanering* (Personnel Planning), PA-rådet, Stockholm 1966.

Bibliography

The organisation theory used as a basis for this study is described in:

Rhenman, E., *The Organisation—A Controlled System*, Stockholm 1966 (SIAR-1).

Rhenman, E., *Industrial Democracy and Industrial Management*, van Gorcum & Comp., Assen, and Tavistock, London 1968 (SIAR-8).

Rhenman, E., *Organization Theory for long-range Planning*, Wiley, London 1973 (SIAR-18).

Rhenman, E., and Stymne, B., *Företagsledning i en föränderlig värld* (Management in a Changing World), Aldus, Stockholm 1965.

Some well-known descriptions of hospitals based on completely different theoretical approaches are:

Argyris, C., *Diagnosing Human Relations in Organizations—A Case Study of a Hospital*, Studies in organizational behavior no. 2, Labor and Management Center, Yale University, New Haven 1956 (mimeograph).

Caudill, W., *The Psychiatric Hospital as a Small Society*, Harvard University Press, Cambridge Mass. 1958.

Coser, R. L.,'Authority and Decision-making in a Hospital: A Comparative Analysis' *American Sociological Review*, 23:1, 1958, pp. 56-63.

Dunham, H., and Weinberg, S. K., *The Culture of the State Mental Hospital*, Wayne-State University Press, Detroit 1960.

Freidson, E. (ed.), *The Hospital in Modern Society—Eleven Studies of the Hospital Today*, The Free Press of Glencoe, New York 1963.

Georgopoulos, B. S., and Tannenbaum, A. S., 'A Study of Organizational Effectiveness' *American Sociological Review*, 22:5, 1957, pp. 534-540.

Israel, J., *Hur patienten upplever sjukhuset* (How the Patient Feels about the Hospital), Almqvist & Wiksell, Stockholm 1962.

Lawrence, P.R., and Lorsch, J.W., *Organization and Environment. Managing Differentiation and Integration*, Harvard University, Boston 1967.

Perrow, C., *Authority, Goals and Prestige in a General Hospital*, unpublished doctoral thesis, University of California, Berkeley 1960.

Perrow, C., 'The Analysis of Goals in Complex Organizations', *American*

Sociological Review, 26, 1961, pp. 854-866.

Perrow, C., 'Goals and Power Structures–A Historical Case Study', in E. Freidson (ed.), *The Hospital in Modern Society*, The Free Press of Glencoe, New York 1963, pp. 112-146.

Perrow, C.,'Hospitals: Technology, Structure and Goals', in J. March (ed.), *Handbook of Organizations,* Rand McNally, Chicago 1965.

Additional information about Swedish hospitals and medical care with completely different approaches can be obtained from:

Biörck, G., 'Om tio år' (In Ten Years), *Svenska Läkartidningen*, 62:1, 1965, p. 21.

Biörck, G., *'Sjukvårdens villkor. Debattinlägg om läkare, sjuksköterskor och sjukhus* (Conditions for Medical Care. A Contribution to the Debate on Doctors, Nurses and Hospitals), Stockholm 1966.

Biörck, G., 'Ledningsproblem inom sjukvården' (Administrative Problems in Medical Care), in *Samhälle i omvandling*, published in honour of Tore Browaldh's fiftieth birthday, Stockholm 1967.

Biörck, G., Wijnbladh, H., and Lundquist, J. (ed.), 'Inför morgondagens hälso- och sjukvård' (Confronting Tomorrow's Health and Medical Care) *Symposier i Svenska Läkaresällskapet*, Tidens Förlag, Stockholm 1963.

Borgenhammar, E., *Sjukhusets ekonomiska ledning* (Financial Administration of the Hospital), EFI, Stockholm 1967 (mimeograph).

Borgenhammar, E., and Otterland, A.,'Sjukvårdsadministratörernas utbildning' (Education of Hospital Administrators), *Svenska Läkartidningen* 61:18, 1964, p. 1480.

Heimann, P., *Bättre sjukvård* (Improved Medical Care), Bonniers, Stockholm 1964.

En frekvensstudie vid en vårdavdelning–En vårdbehovsanalys, ett. försök att finna ett samband mellan patienternas vårdbehov och personalens arbetsinsats (A Frequency Study in a Clinical Department–An Analysis of Requirements for Care, an Attempt to Find a Link between the Patients' Needs and the Personnel's Efforts), Organisation Bureau, The Central Board of Hospital Planning, Stockholm 1966 (mimeograph).

Läkarjourtjänsten–Omfattningen och karaktären av sjukhusläkarnas jourarbete jämte vissa förslag (Doctors on call–Extent and Nature of Hospital Doctors' On-call Service and Some Proposals), Organisation Department, Swedish Association of County Councils, 1965:10.

Rapport över en studie beträffande personalfunktion och personal-omsättning vid Centrallasarettet i Eskilstuna (Report on a Study of Personnel Functions and Turnover at General Hospital in Eskilstuna), Consultation Department, The Swedish Council for Personnel Administration, Stockholm 1965 (mimeograph).

'Sjukhusläkares arbete och ansvar' (The Work and Responsibility of Hospital Doctors in the USA), study performed by U. Serner, Stockholm 1966.

De statliga undervisningssjukhusens organisation. Betänkande avgivet av 1963 års klinikutredning (The Organisation of State Teaching Hospitals—Report presented by the Clinical Study of 1963), SOU, no. 37, Stockholm 1966.

Index

Indexer's note: in this index, where a specific item is not shown, please see under *hospital* when it refers only to the hospital investigated, and under *hospitals* when it refers to hospitals as a whole.

300

302

303